NEVER FEAR FALLING AGAIN

SIMPLE AND EASY EXERCISES FOR FALL PREVENTION
YOU CAN PERFORM AT HOME AND FEEL SAFER IN 28
DAYS - WITH EXCLUSIVE READER ACCESS TO
EXERCISE VIDEOS

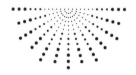

KOOROSH NAGHSHINEH, PH.D.

SELF-PUBLISHED

Dedication

To my parents, who supported me all my life and were always there for me, even over long distances.

THANK YOU

This book would not have been possible without the loving support and participation of my beautiful wife, Linda. Without her help in checking the exercises, helping me make the exercise photos and videos, and editing, this book would not have been possible.

I am indebted to my daughter, Leila, for suggesting that I write. This is the first book I have written. Her support and encouragement has always been a blessing in my life.

In addition, I am always grateful for my daughter Mimi and her support in anything I get myself into.

Finally, I am thankful for the help of my friends and colleagues, Jim and Massoud, in reviewing this book and suggesting revisions.

TABLE OF CONTENTS

HOW THIS BOOK CAME ABOUT

It was one morning in November 2019, my phone buzzed. I had a text from my brother. "Mom just broke her leg, I am waiting for the ambulance!!" This was the start of a series of terrible events in my mother's life. Because of her severe osteoporosis, her femur had broken close to the hip joint. She did't fall. She was just putting on her clothes when this happened. She went through an operation and a long recovery. A few months later she recovered enough to be able to walk with the help of a cane. Because she knew she had a severe case of osteoporosis, she was now extremely afraid of falling down. Turns out this is a fear faced by many seniors.

Sadly, this was not the end of my mother's problems. Shortly after she was mobile again, she experienced the same problem in her other leg. The same bone had broken in her other leg at the same spot! Again she went through a long process of surgery, recovery, and rehabilitation. Her fears of falling down became even worse than before. This prohibited her from being active. Today she is bound to using her walker all the time and feels very limited about her choice of activities.

My goal in writing this book is to help you stay active and mobile. No one should be crippled by fear of such injuries. With the right tools and guidance, independence and vitality can be preserved. This book is for those willing to work for their freedom of movement and enjoy the later years of life without crippling fear.

To have an active life in your later years, you need to make sure you have good balance. To have good balance you need strong core muscles. You need to keep moving and stay active. All of this requires you to exercise. This book provides you with a set of exercises that can help you improve your balance. I present you with a wide variety of exercises. Start where you can and build up. Make sure to involve your physician. The last thing I want is for you to injure yourself. Have a conversation with your doctor and make sure you know what exercises are safe for you.

I am a retired Mechanical Engineering professor so I tend to think through problems very systematically. I like learning and teaching. I have been an exercise enthusiast since I was a teenager. To this day, I walk a few miles a day, lift weights, and play tennis and pickle-ball when I can. My exercise habits have changed as I have gotten older. Every morning I perform a set of stretches (similar to what you see in this book) that help me feel free of aches and pains I wake up with. This also keeps me active. In this book, I am sharing some of what I have learned and experienced. I wish I could have provided this material to my mother long ago. I hope that you will find this book helpful.

FREE GIFTS FOR THE READER

Thank you for reading *Never Fear Falling Again*. I hope you will find it insightful, inspiring, and most importantly practical. I hope it helps you build a strong and healthy body with excellent balance so you can feel safe and confident as you enjoy your life.

To help you get the best results as fast as possible, I have included the following additional bonus materials at no extra cost to you. These are:

- ***Videos of the exercises listed in this book. These videos show you how you can do these exercises at home.***
- A chapter-by-chapter list of all exercises along with the photos.
- A weekly exercise planner.

To get your bonuses, please scan this image using your cell-phone camera.

Alternatively, you can go to this link:

https://www.betterbalanceforall.com

In both cases, you will be directed to the same website where you will create an account and receive access to this material. My goal is to continue to add useful material to this website to help you succeed in improving your health and balance.

INTRODUCTION

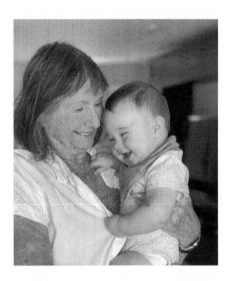

The long-awaited retirement stage of life has finally come. For some, reaching this stage is met with joy and relief. For others, this stage of life might be a bit intimidating, due to physical instability and a fear of falling. When imagining retirement, time spent with grand-children and taking up new hobbies comes to mind. But if a fear of falling prevents one from doing these things, retirement can be frustrating and even lonely.

The good news is that there are actions you can take to regain your confidence and enjoy being physically active again in just 28 days. It is common for seniors to avoid doing the things they once loved due to instability, pain, and loss of stamina. Thankfully, this doesn't have to be the case. It is never too late to rebuild muscle strength, and it doesn't take vigorous gym exercises to achieve results. It is also never too early to take action. Even if you do not have balance problems, you can, and you should, have a regular exercise program similar to what is described in this book

To address physical limitations associated with the fear of falling, this book will cover topics such as **common causes of balance problems** including one associated with the flu, how to fight off dizziness without having to take medications, what system acts as the body's stabilizer, and how to enhance this area and improve posture. It will go over the **five major benefits of stretching** and give a thorough explanation of the system responsible for maintaining balance and control. We'll talk about **how to prepare the body for stretching** so that maximum benefits can be achieved, with a number of detailed exercises that will contribute to increased strength and stability. Included is **the number one exercise that can improve balance** without the high risk of injury. To address delayed exercise soreness, there is an added ten minute activity that will reduce pain and inflammation. Also included are **outlines of effective weekly exercise plans** for life-changing results in just 28 days.

To address the mental limitations associated with the fear of falling, *Never Fear Falling Again* will present facts that **debunk six myths about exercising and aging**. The unknown often leads to fear, but if a light is shined before us, confidence is restored, work to move forward can be done, and progress is made.

The facts, science, stretches, and exercises presented here will combine to give readers all the necessary tools to live an active and pain-free life well into their senior years. Retirement can be a haven of lasting memories made just as we expect it to be.

Choosing to digest and apply the knowledge provided here is the first step toward a stronger body and a fruitful life. Every day gives us something beautiful to enjoy: a walk in the park with the family, a vacation with loved ones, or time spent doing the things that give us happiness and joy. Using this book to improve your health and wellness will empower you to live a new life with deeper love and many wonderful memories to come.

Start savoring what life has to offer by overcoming the fear of falling and equipping the body to be stronger, more flexible, and more stable by following the **S**tretching, **M**obility, and **M**uscle strength (SMM approach) provided here.

HOW TO USE THIS BOOK

This book has two goals. The first is to educate you about the importance of balance and how it can be affected by many factors. The second is to provide you with an array of exercises that will help you improve your balance.

As you will see, many exercises are described in this book. At my count, there are:

- Chapter 2: 17 Seated exercises
- Chapter 3: 18 Standing exercises
- Chapter 4: 11 Core exercises
- Chapter 5: 20 Stretching exercises
- Chapter 6: 36 Inner ear and vestibular exercises
- Chapter 7: 6 Arthritis exercises
- Chapter 8: 5 Tai Chi exercises

At first glance, this may be overwhelming. How do you decide which exercise to start with?

My recommendation is that you start with the exercises in Chapter 2. If you feel that you can easily master these exercises, move on to the exercises in Chapter 3. Once you have mastered the exercises in Chapter 3, move on to the ones in

Chapter 4. You need a strong core (through Chapter 4) to have good balance.

Although I have described a few stretching exercises in Chapters 2 and 3, Chapter 5 focuses entirely on stretching exercises. These can be adopted to help you warm up before or cool down after doing the exercises in the other chapters.

Once you have mastered all the exercises through Chapter 5, you can pick and choose your own favorites. This doesn't mean you will choose the easiest exercises :) What I am asking you to do is to find the exercises you find challenging and focus on those until you have mastered them. What does it mean to master an exercise? It means you have done it enough times, that over time, it can be done without struggle. Typically, exercises practiced for four weeks (28 days) will start to show benefits. Make sure to include some stretching exercises before and after your program.

For those readers who suffer from inner ear problems causing dizziness or those who suffer from arthritis, I have devoted a chapter (Chapter 6) to exercises addressing each of these issues. The exercises in Chapter 6 are described but not illustrated. My focus was to make you familiar with these exercises but to have you only perform these exercises in the presence of a trained professional practitioner. Thus, I did not include any illustrations of these exercises.

A few specialized exercises are described in Chapters 7 and 8. You can do these on your own or sign up for a class where you will be guided deeper into these types of exercises. Finally, Chapter 9 is entirely devoted to dealing with the after effects of exercise and how to deal with muscle soreness.

In order to help you better follow the instructions provided in this book, where possible, I have recorded **videos demonstrating the exercises mentioned in this book**. You can gain access to these videos by registering at our website (www.betterbalanceforall.com). I hope that you can take advantage of these videos since they will enhance your understanding of the exercises.

Never Fear Falling Again will guide you every step of the way!

1
WHAT IS BALANCE?

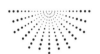

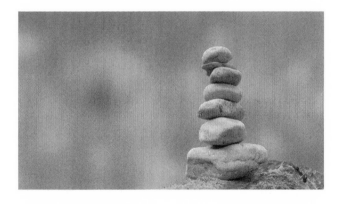

Falls are resulting in over 3 million injuries per year and lead to over 800,000 hospitalizations in the United States.

Doing balance improving exercises regularly can prevent falls and promote enjoyable activities the senior years have to offer. Balancing exercises have an array of added benefits and are necessary to maintain stability and confidence.

But have you ever wondered... What *is* balance, exactly? What factors affect it?

Balance is the ability to maintain even weight distribution to stand upright and remain steady on our feet. Balance is something that we grow into developmentally within the first years of life. As the **three systems that control balance** mature, we become more stable and confident in our physical activities. These systems include **vision**, **proprioception** (how our body senses its position in space), and **the inner ear** or vestibular system. **The vestibular system** stabilizes our vision when the head moves.

The importance of improving all three systems is emphasized throughout this book, because it is the cooperation and coordination of the three that leads to the greatest stability and balance. Also, if one system cannot function at full capacity for any reason (such as deteriorating eyesight) then the other two systems may compensate to maintain stability and control (K. McIntyre, 2022).

WHY YOU NEED TO DO BALANCE EXERCISES

Balancing exercises are necessary for the later years of life for a multitude of reasons, including maintaining stability. They decrease the risk of falling by increasing muscle mass and overall strength, improving cognitive function, and promoting more restful sleep. They also improve reaction times, strengthen bones, and enhance coordination. The collective benefits of doing balancing exercises result in gained confidence, agility, and stamina.

Even if you do not have a current balance problem, you should perform the exercises in this book (or any similar exercises) in order to maintain your health and assure yourself of good balance in your future.

SIX MYTHS ABOUT EXERCISING AND AGING

Myth One: "Since I'm getting old anyway, there's no reason to exercise."

Fact: The truth is, we're all getting older and that shouldn't hold us back from exercising. Physical activity keeps us agile, strong, and encourages mental positivity. It also helps protect against some of the most common conditions that become more prevalent as we age such as dementia and Alzheimer's, some cancers, obesity, diabetes, and certain heart conditions.

Myth Two: "If I exercise then I'm more likely to fall."

Fact: Exercising regularly helps to build up muscle mass, agility, and improves stamina. All of these benefits will help to maintain stability and control, lowering the risk of falling.

Myth Three: "Knowing I'll never be as athletic as I once was makes exercise too discouraging."

Fact: It's important to be kind and understanding of the natural life cycle. Yes, it is true that our most athletic years present at an earlier age. But staying active and physically fit later in life is admirable and something anyone can be proud of. The fact is that remaining sedentary will deteriorate an athletic body faster than aging will.

Myth Four: *"It's too late for me to start exercising."*

Fact: No one is ever too old to begin an exercise routine and start living a healthier life. Starting an exercise program later in life will show more immediate and greater improvements in mood and physical fitness than starting at a younger age. One benefit of only starting to become active in the senior years is that there won't be any old sports injuries to flare-up and cause trouble. The key is to start slow and set reasonable goals.

Myth Five: *"Being disabled means I can't exercise."*

Fact: Certain accommodations need to be made if you're a person with disabilities, but exercise is still possible and beneficial. Several routines can be modified to focus on the areas of the body that are not affected by a disability. Strength training and swimming are a couple of examples of physical activities that can be adjusted to most physical limitations.

Myth Six: *"I am not strong enough or am too sore to exercise."*

Fact: Staying mobile and active will help reduce aches and pains, as well as build up muscle strength. Regular exercise will help reverse the muscle deterioration that comes with aging, and result in more enjoyable later years of life. Just remember to start slowly and the muscles will build up in no time.

COMMON CAUSES OF BALANCE PROBLEMS

Medication Side Effects

Several medications are commonly prescribed to the elderly that contribute to the loss of balance. Some of these drugs are intended to lower blood pressure which can result in dizziness and lightheadedness. Antidepressants, sedatives, and some cancer-treating medications can result in fatigue making it harder to exercise to maintain muscle strength. Being sleepy can make anyone accident prone, so there's no wonder why these types of medications can be a contributing factor to one's risk of falling. Make sure to discuss possible side effects of your medications with your physician.

Meniere's Disease

Meniere's disease affects the inner ear and can result in feeling as though the ears are filled with water. As stated by the National Institutes of Health (NIH), some instances of the disease can lead to vertigo, loss of hearing, and decreased balance. However, it can be treated with medication, a specialized low-sodium diet, and the balance training provided in this book.

If there is suspicion that Meniere's disease could be contributing to the loss of balance, then a physician should be consulted for proper treatment.

Vision–Related Problems

Deterioration of the eyes as we age lends itself to several common vision problems, such as cataracts and macular degeneration. Regular visits to the ophthalmologist are highly recommended to maintain the best vision possible. Some conditions can be reversed while others can be treated and the effects greatly minimized.

Chronic Conditions

According to the NIH, studies are showing a relationship between diabetes and vestibular dysfunction which ultimately lead to a reduced sense of balance. Other chronic conditions that can also affect balance and stability include chronically high blood pressure, recurring thyroid disorders, heart disease, and arthritis. Some medical conditions that compromise the central nervous system and contribute to instability are multiple sclerosis, Alzheimer's disease, and Parkinson's disease.

If any of these conditions are suspected then a physician should be sought out for proper treatment. If balance and stability are being affected by any of these conditions, talking to a physician about further options is encouraged.

Benign Paroxysmal Positioning Vertigo (BPPV)

BPPV can cause intense spinning sensation which can result in balance problems. It causes periods of dizziness that can follow mild physical activities such as getting out of bed or standing up from a seated position. Treatment options include head movement exercises that can help manage symptoms.

A physician should be immediately consulted if one is experiencing any signs of vertigo.

Labyrinthitis

This inner ear infection can be responsible for loss of balance due to the disruption of nerve signals that commute from the inner ear to the brain. This infection is associated with severe cases of the flu and is, therefore, more common in the senior population.

Seeking treatment from a physician is highly recommended and will entail both medicinal treatments as well as some recommended physical activity alterations to reduce vertigo episodes.

Age-Related Hearing Loss

Presbycusis, or age-related hearing loss, accumulates over time and is often not noticed immediately by the individual presenting symptoms. Unfortunately, hearing loss can be a result of bone, blood vessel, or tissue changes and can impact one's balance.

A person's quality of hearing should be regularly assessed by a physician, and if hearing loss is found, treatment options may include hearing aids or other devices.

Poor Circulation

In the later years of life, the blood vessels are not quite as effective as they once were. This can cause blood to move more slowly through the body and result in insufficient oxygen supply to the brain after a quick movement. For example, when standing too quickly, the blood pressure drops and can lead to a spell of dizziness or lightheadedness that could cause a loss of balance and potential fall.

Consult a physician if low blood pressure is a concern, as it could be from poor circulation or medication, and should be addressed immediately.

CONFIRMATION THAT BALANCE IS A PROBLEM

Let's first confirm that balance truly is an issue. Everyone can lose their balance from time to time, but if the occurrence is frequent or causes fear and a withdrawal from enjoying activities, then there may be some work to do to restore strength, confidence, and stability.

Ask yourself the following questions from the National Institute on Aging to determine if you're experiencing balance issues beyond that of a normal occurrence.

If the answer to any of these questions is "yes" then talk to a physician about what could be causing the issue and possible mitigations that can be taken before starting a new exercise program.

- Do I ever feel unsteady?
- Do I feel as if the room is spinning at times, even if it is only for a few moments?
- Do I feel as if I'm moving even when I know my body is still?
- Do I ever lose my balance and fall?
- Do I ever feel as though I'm falling even when I know I'm not?
- Do I ever feel lightheaded, or like I might faint?
- Do I ever experience blurry vision?
- Do I ever feel disoriented, lose the sense of time, place, or identity?

(NIH National Institute on Aging, 2017)

If a balance issue is confirmed and a physician has approved balance and stretching exercises to improve stability, continue to the next chapter for the start of a journey leading to confidence, balance, and strength. The seated exercises are presented first in this guide, and can be performed in the home without any specialized equipment. The key to succeeding in any new journey is taking the next step. *Never Fear Falling Again* will lead the way.

2

SEATED EXERCISES

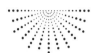

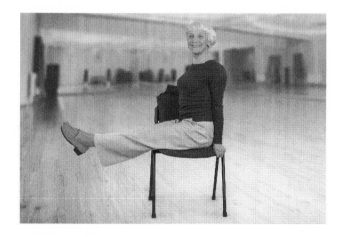

A common misunderstanding is that exercising means intense physical activity. This is not always the case, and certainly not necessary for the movements outlined in this chapter.

These exercises are perfect for someone who needs the added stability of a chair, and allow for full participation while fully supported. They are a perfect start for anyone fearing injury from a fall and improve muscle strength and joint mobility for better balance.

The benefits of seated exercises include a greater range of motion and flexibility, reduced pain and stiffness in the joints, strengthening of the muscles, improved blood circulation, reduced stress, and endorphin release for an uplift in mood. For all of these reasons, seated exercises are a wonderful option for those looking to get fit without risking a fall or injury.

We'll begin with warm-up motions before moving into arm and leg exercises to do over the next 28 days. Then add a bit of aerobics to get the heart pumping, and end the routine with some stretching for improving flexibility and preventing muscle soreness. So, let's get started!

WARM-UP EXERCISES

Regardless of age or physical ability, exercise should always be preceded by a warm-up and stretch of the muscles to prevent injury. The warm-ups provided are perfect for seniors to do from a seated position, and will contribute to greater motion without pain during the exercises to follow.

It's also important for you to be conscious of your breathing. Exhale as you lift a weight, inhale as you relax and lower the weights. During stretches, focus on slow and controlled breathing.

NECK STRETCH

With the back straight and the body in a neutral sitting position, gently turn your head to the right to align the chin with the shoulder. Don't worry if limited mobility prevents full alignment of the chin and shoulder. Allow for a gentle stretch in the neck while reaching downward with the left hand. Hold this position for a few moments and then repeat it on the other side. Repeat the stretch two to five times on each side until the muscles in the neck and upper back feel warm and loose.

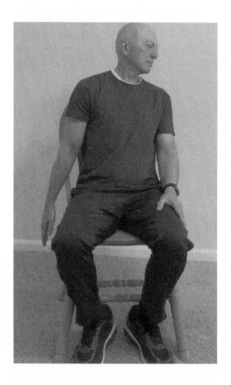

SHOULDER CIRCLES

Place the fingertips of each hand on the corresponding shoulder and rotate the shoulder forward 15 times. Repeat this stretch rotating the shoulder backward another 15 times. This warm-up will loosen up the muscles in the shoulders and allow for greater movement without pain.

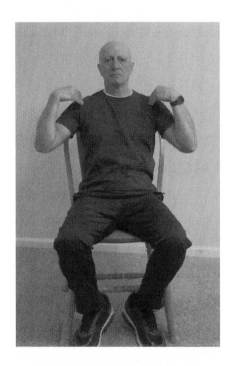

CHAIR EXERCISES FOR ARMS

Muscle mass deteriorates with inactivity, which is why it is so important to do some amount of exercise regularly. With greater strength comes greater stability and confidence to move through daily activities without falling. Strength directly contributes to one's independence and sense of freedom. Notice the improved strength the next time a grandchild is lifted for a hug. Enjoy the benefits of stronger arms with only three short exercises provided here.

Bicep Curls

Resistance bands or small weights (can even be two cans of soup) can be used for the bicep curl and each should be chosen with the appropriate level of difficulty. If using resistance bands, place the feet on top of the band shoulder-width apart and grip the handles with the elbows close to the torso. Begin the bicep curl using the feet to secure the band to the floor. Bring the gripped handles up to the shoulders slowly and then back down to align with the thigh. It is important to keep the elbows tucked inward at all times and use only the bicep to curl upward. If using weights, repeat the same motion with the upward arm curl with the feet firmly planted on the floor. Move through this exercise slowly and at your own pace for three sets of ten repetitions.

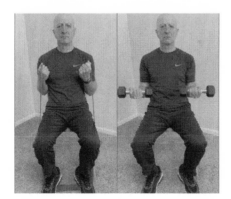

SEATED ROW

While seated toward the front of your seat, with feet planted firmly to the ground, extend the arms forward with thumbs pointing upward. Using the back muscles to pull the shoulder blades together, gradually move your elbows backward until they align with the torso. Repeat this exercise extending arms back out and squeezing the upper back while moving the elbows to align with the torso another eight to ten times. Wrist weights can be used for this exercise when you're ready for the added challenge.

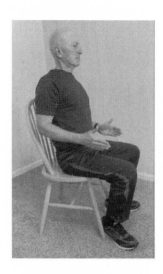

SHOULDER ROLLS

While sitting up straight with the feet firmly planted on the ground, pull the shoulders up towards the ears and then rotate them slowly in a full circle. Repeat the shoulder roll going forwards and backward ten times each. This exercise will strengthen the muscles responsible for lifting and carrying.

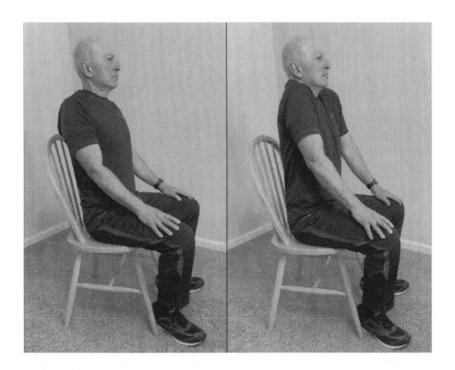

CHAIR EXERCISES FOR LEGS

There is a common misconception that leg exercises cannot be done while seated. Toe taps and knee lifts are perfect exercises to perform from the comfort and stability of a chair and will contribute to overall strength in the legs for greater mobility and stamina.

TOE TAPS

Begin with a straight back and feet planted on the ground. Lift the toes upward off the ground while keeping the heel of each foot planted and then return the toes back to the ground. Repeat this exercise eight to ten times. For a greater challenge, sit toward the front of the chair and extend the legs straight with just the heels on the ground. Flex the toes back toward the body and then forward again. This exercise will strengthen the calf and shin muscles that are used often in daily activities and when climbing stairs.

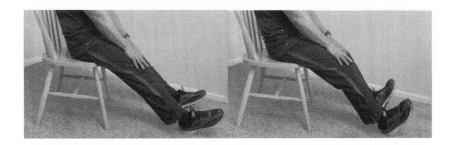

KNEE LIFTS

While sitting upright with a straight back and feet flat on the ground, slowly raise one knee toward the chest, count to five, and then return the foot gently to the ground again. Repeat this knee lift on each leg for a total of 20 repetitions. Add ankle weights if more of a challenge is desired. Knee lifts strengthen the quad muscles and will provide added stability in everyday activities.

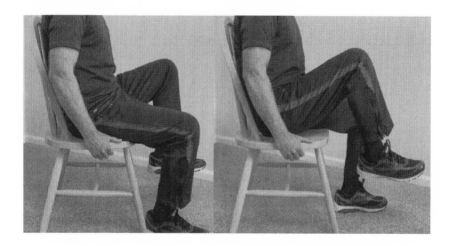

CORE EXERCISES

Core exercises are essential for maintaining balance and stability. The exercises outlined below are intended to strengthen the critical muscle group for seniors that will assist in preventing falls. They focus on working the muscles in the lower back, abs, and glutes. The core muscles are the foundation from which we can stay active and mobile. The Tummy Twist and Captain's Chair are perfect for targeting these muscle groups.

TUMMY TWISTS

While seated upright with a straight back and feet planted firmly on the floor, cross your arms at shoulder level (the "I Dream of a Jeanie" pose). Turn the entire torso to the right with the stomach firm and engaged. Ensure that the lower portion of the body remains still. Turn slowly back to center and repeat the twist to the right a total of ten times before doing the same to the left. This exercise will contribute to better posture, strengthen obliques and abdominals, and improve overall balance.

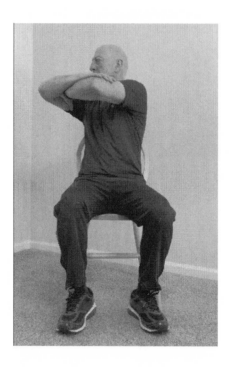

Captain's Chair

Perform this exercise from a chair that is stable on the ground and has comfortably strong arms for grasping. Begin by sitting with a straight back, holding onto the chair, and raising the feet off of the floor to bring the knees close to the chest. If you don't have an arm chair, grasp the two sides of the chair. Be sure to engage the stomach muscles and move slowly. Return the feet to the floor. Even if only able to raise the feet just off the floor, this exercise will strengthen the core with time and practice. Start with five repetitions and increase to as many as you can (and as high off the floor as you can).

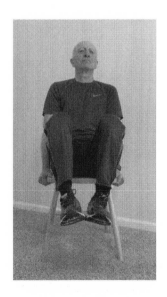

CHAIR AEROBICS FOR CARDIO

Cardio exercises focus on strengthening the heart and contribute to better circulation and blood flow. They also reduce the risk of heart attack and improve stamina during everyday activities. These exercises will also expand lung capacity and allow for easier breathing during physical activity.

Seated Jumping Jacks

This exercise is ideally performed when seated in an armless chair but can be modified with careful awareness when performed in a chair with arms as well. While sitting upright with a straight back, extend the arms with a straight elbow downward at the side of the body. Move the arms quickly upward as though performing a standing jumping jack. Repeat this motion as quickly as possible 20 times. Note that the speed of this exercise will improve over time and with practice.

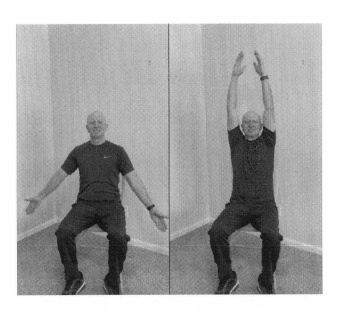

Skater Switch

While sitting towards the front of the chair, straighten the left leg out and slightly to the side, while keeping a pointed toe. Start with both arms extended out in front of the body, and then reach the left hand down toward the right foot, with the right arm extending backward. Come back up with both arms out in front of the body and repeat the motion at a speed that is quick but comfortable. Repeat this exercise on each side ten times. Start slow. For an added challenge, alternate reaching to the left and then right more quickly (as safely as possible) while changing the leg position between repetitions.

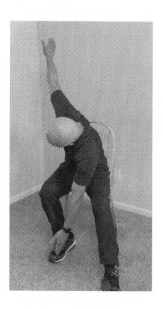

Seated Running

Sit toward the front of the chair, extend the legs out and the arms resting at your sides, lean the shoulders back to gently touch the chair. Then slowly raise the feet from the floor and flex one knee toward the chest while keeping the other straight. Alternate knees in this exercise as though you were running. Use the armrests or the base of the chair to grip for added stability during this exercise. Start with sixty seconds of this exercise or as long as possible and increase the time and how high you bring the feet off the floor as you feel more confident.

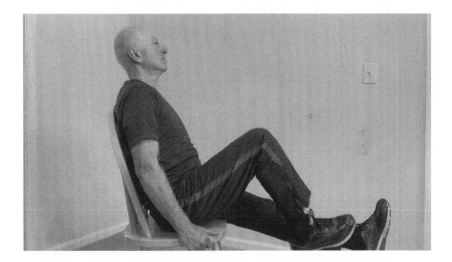

SEATED TAP DANCE

Begin this exercise by sitting upright in a chair with the toes resting gently on the ground. Reach one leg out to tap the heel on the floor. Then point the toes and tap them to the floor before returning the leg to the neutral and bent position. Now switch legs and repeat the steps on the opposite leg. When first starting this exercise, begin doing it for about three minutes or as long as possible. After a week or two, try to increase the time of the exercise to four or five minutes.

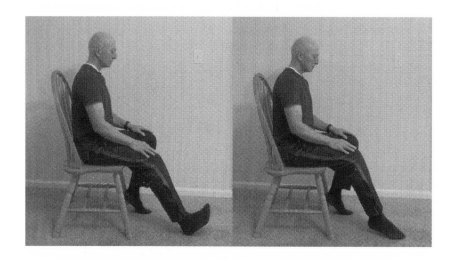

SEATED CHAIR EXERCISES FOR FLEXIBILITY

Increasing flexibility results in greater mobility, less pain, and a wider range of physical abilities. Performing these exercises regularly will allow for exercises to be accomplished at higher levels and for longer durations. Progression in the length and duration of the exercises will result in a stronger body that can enjoy daily activities and empower one to lead their fullest life.

Seated Forward Bend

This exercise begins with open legs and feet planted on the ground. Then lean forward and gently bring the upper body closer to the thighs, while gently stretching your hands toward your feet. Keep the neck loose and hold the position for a few moments, before slowly raising the torso back into a neutral seated position. Perform this stretch three times and notice that with practice flexibility improves. And, don't forget to breathe evenly while stretching.

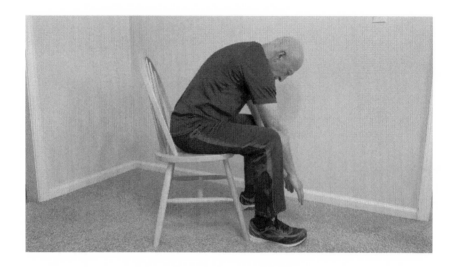

KNEE TO CHEST

Start with an upright posture and the right foot planted on the floor. Support the front of the left knee with your hands and gently pull it inward until a stretch can be felt in the back of the thigh. Hold this stretch for about 30 seconds and return to a neutral position. Repeat this exercise for each leg three times to loosen the hamstrings and glutes. Gaining and maintaining flexibility in these muscles aids in preventing injuries and improving balance.

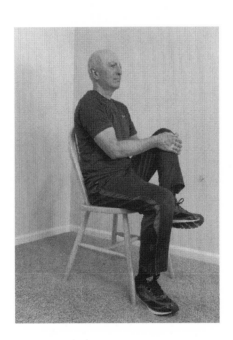

ANKLE ROTATIONS

Starting this exercise, sit tall in a chair with both feet planted firmly on the ground. Now bring one foot off the ground. Move the foot around in a clockwise direction. Then reverse this motion and repeat each direction ten times. For added stretch, point the toes while performing this exercise.

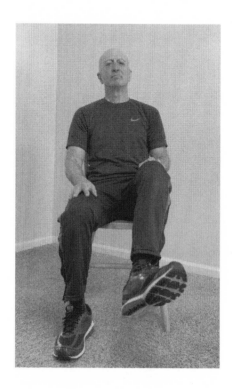

Sit and Reach

In a stable chair, begin this stretch with a straight back and knees together. Raise one arm toward the sky and reach upward to feel a stretch along the side of your torso. To also feel a stretch in the neck and shoulders, turn your head upward towards your hand. Hold this pose for five to ten seconds and then repeat on the opposite side. Repeat the stretch three times on each side.

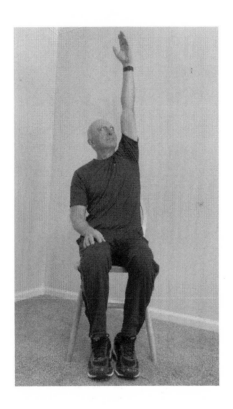

WEEKLY EXERCISE PLAN

The exercises provided in this section include recommended repetitions and timeframes but everyone will start at a slightly different level. There is no need to overdo it. Be gentle with yourself and know that with time there will be significant progress. I encourage you to stop after each exercise (or stretch) to "feel" your body's response.

Consult your primary physician to determine a good starting point for your current fitness level.

An example of a weekly chair exercise plan is outlined below and may seem like a lot but feel free to break the day's workout into sections. If you get tired, take a rest, and come back to the other exercises later. The goal is for you to perform four weeks of these exercises and build your strength by moving every day.

If at any point you're experiencing pain, consult a physician immediately.

See videos of these exercises at www.betterbalanceforall.com

* * *

SAMPLE SEATED EXERCISE PLAN

Monday: Seated Warm-Up Exercises , Chair Exercises for Arms, Chair Core Exercises

Tuesday: Chair Exercises for Legs, Chair Aerobics, Chair Flexibility Exercises

Wednesday: Seated Warm-Up Exercises , Chair Exercises for Arms, Chair Aerobics, Chair Core Exercises

Thursday: Chair Core Exercises and Chair Flexibility Exercises

Friday: Seated Warm-Up Exercises , Chair Aerobics, Chair Flexibility Exercises

Saturday: Chair Aerobics, Warm-Up Chair Exercises, Chair Core Exercises, Chair Flexibility Exercises

Sunday: Seated Warm-Up Exercises , Chair Core Exercises, Chair Flexibility Exercises

Seated exercises will allow for progress, even if it is in small increments. Every day will get a bit easier with the muscles being conditioned and loosened daily. When you're ready, try standing exercises to continue to build on strength and balance. See the next chapter to discover how to perform them.

3

STANDING EXERCISES

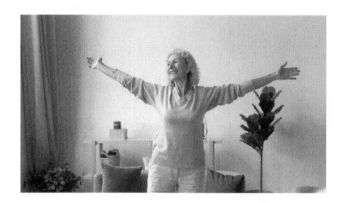

M ost falls are a result of walking or standing, so
it is important to establish balance in an
upright position. Building strength and agility
will contribute to an overall better sense of balance and
increased stamina.

Consult a physician to determine if you're ready for standing
exercises before proceeding with this chapter.

When you begin the standing exercises, go at a pace that is right for you. We'll suggest durations and repetitions of the exercises but know that if you're unable to complete it, that's okay. By continuing to do your best, the muscles will become stronger and the exercises will become easier to complete. Enjoy these standing exercises as you journey towards your next level of strongest self over the next 28 days.

EXERCISES

Single-Leg Stance

To perform this exercise, begin by standing next to a chair or countertop that can be used as a stabilizer. While holding onto the chair or countertop, lift one leg slightly off the floor while bending the knee at a comfortable angle. Maintain good posture and an engaged core to optimize the improved balance benefits of this exercise. Hold the pose with the leg lifted for seconds before returning it to the ground. Five to ten seconds is good but it's up to you as to how long you can hold this pose safely. Repeat this exercise five times on each leg.

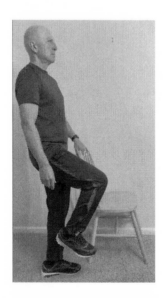

For added balance support, use both hands to brace yourself on a chair or countertop. As your balance improves, these exercises can be performed without the use of a stabilizer. This particular exercise is extremely important because it mimics walking and stair climbing. These activities are the primary culprits of trips and fall when one loses balance. Strengthening all of the muscles involved will improve walking and climbing capabilities.

FOOT TAPS TO STEP

Beginning with a straight back, face a step. Use a chair or railing to stabilize during the exercise if necessary. Slowly raise one foot off of the ground to tap the step in front of you and then return the foot to the floor. Maintain good posture and an engaged core while performing this exercise. Avoid swinging the leg by moving slowly and in a controlled manner. Tap each foot to the step ten times each and repeat the exercise on each leg two to three times. Foot taps improve the muscle coordination used when climbing the stairs and help in preventing trips and falls.

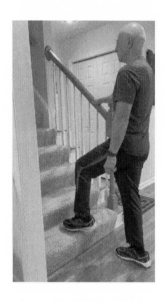

Narrow Stance Reaches

Start this exercise by placing the feet as close together as possible while maintaining a stable stance. Reach one or both hands out in front of the body and then return them, with bent elbows, inward towards the body in a slow and controlled motion. A stabilizer can be used with this exercise while one arm reaches forward as well. If you're ready for a bit of a challenge and do not need a stabilizer, reach the arms straight out in front of the body and then out to the sides before bending the elbows to bring them back in. Repeat this exercise ten times. This exercise improves the ability to reach out for an item in a tight space and trains the core to balance the body.

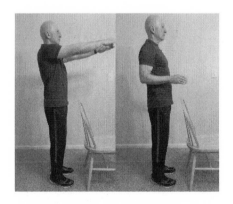

3-WAY HIP KICK

This exercise is performed while holding onto a chair or countertop to maintain balance and control. Start by lifting the foot out in front of the body with a straight leg. It is okay if you can only lift it slightly off the floor. After a moment, return the foot to the floor in a controlled motion. Then lift the leg out to the side and after a moment return the foot back to the floor. Next, lift the leg to the back and bring the foot back to the floor. Repeat this exercise five to ten times on each leg for one repetition. Perform two to three repetitions on each leg. The 3-way hip kick will improve strength and flexibility in the hips and will ease activities such as walking, climbing stairs, and turning around.

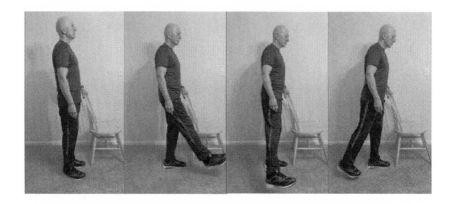

STANDING MARCHES

Use a chair or tabletop to stabilize the body while performing this exercise. Hold onto the stabilizer and raise one knee to a 90-degree angle or as high as you're able. Hold this stance for a moment before returning the foot to the ground. Repeat this motion 20 times for a single repetition on one leg before switching to the other leg. Each leg should perform two to three repetitions. If looking to increase the difficulty of this exercise, try stabilizing the body with only one hand or removing the stabilizer altogether. Standing marches will improve the body's ability to respond quickly if tripping to step out and catch oneself. They improve balance and hip strength as well.

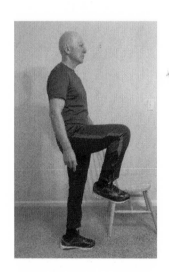

MINI LUNGES

With or without a chair to assist with stabilizing, begin this exercise with the feet about shoulder-width apart. Step forward with the front knee bent slightly and then step back into the starting position. Repeat the mini lunge on each leg ten times. Be sure to use a chair or countertop to hold onto if you're experiencing any knee or hip pain. Also, this exercise can be modified by taking a shallower step forward when performing the mini lunge. This exercise also assists with catching yourself if you trip. It also aids in strengthening the leg muscles for improved stamina.

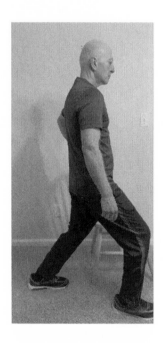

LATERAL STEPPING

To perform this exercise, start by standing with the feet together, then step to the side just wider than the width of the shoulders. Step the foot back toward the center in a controlled motion. Repeat this exercise five to ten times for repetition before switching to the other leg. Perform two to three repetitions per leg. For added stability, hold onto a chair or countertop. The lateral step improves coordination with stepping and turning a small space and assists in avoiding loss of balance under these circumstances.

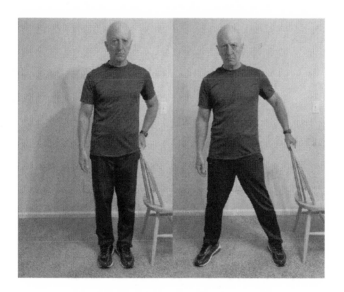

Squats

While standing with the feet about shoulder-width apart, bend down in a sitting motion as far as you comfortably (and safely) are able to. Hold onto a chair or countertop to avoid falling if necessary. Squat ten times, take a short break and repeat another ten squats two more times. Squats strengthen the glutes and thigh muscles to improve balance and agility when standing from a seated position. Squat down only as far as you can comfortably stand back up. Your range of motion will increase with practice.

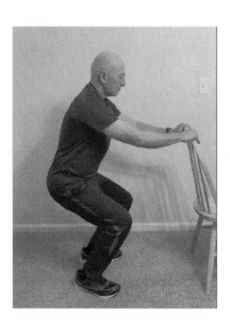

TANDEM OR SEMI-TANDEM STANCE

Perform this exercise using a table or chair to stabilize if necessary. Begin by stepping the right foot in front of the left so that the heel of the right foot aligns with the toe of the left. Try to avoid a gap between the feet as much as possible and hold the position for ten seconds. Return the right foot beside the left and repeat the exercise two to three times before performing the same on the opposite side. This position naturally puts the body into a tight space while exercising muscles that keep you stabilized.

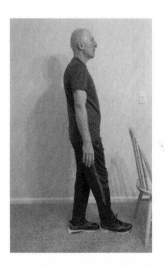

As your balance improves, try to perform the Tandem Stance without holding onto a chair or table. If the Tandem Stance is too difficult for you, you can set one foot in front of the other foot with a slight gap in between your feet. This is called the Semi-Tandem Stance.

Heel Raises

While standing with the feet shoulder-width apart, raise the heels off of the ground while shifting your weight to the balls of your feet. Then slowly return the heels to the ground. Repeat this exercise ten times for one repetition and perform two to three total repetitions. Heel raises strengthen the calf muscles and ankle muscles to improve overall balance when standing and walking.

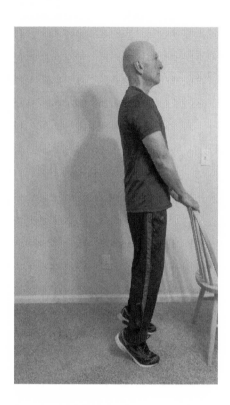

HAMSTRING STRETCH

Begin this exercise by holding on to a chair and placing the heel of one foot on the ground out in front of you. Gently bend the body toward the foot and hold for ten to 20 seconds. Repeat this stretch on each leg two to three times. Hamstrings can become especially tight from sitting for long periods. The hamstring stretch loosens the hamstring muscles for better agility and decreased cramping when walking and standing.

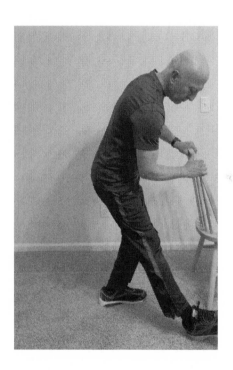

CALF STRETCH

Holding onto a countertop or leaning on a wall works best for the calf stretch. Step one foot slightly forward, keeping the heel braced on the ground and placing the toe of the foot against the base of the counter. Move the body forward slightly until a gentle stretch can be felt in the calf muscle and hold the position for 10–20 seconds. Return the body to an upright position and repeat on the opposite leg. Repeat this exercise on each leg two to three times. Calf stretches prevent cramps and soreness.

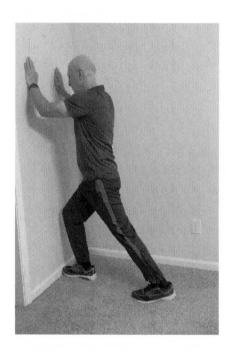

Head Rotation

Start in a comfortable standing position and begin this stretch by turning the head from left to right, then nodding up and down. Be sure to keep movements slow and controlled to avoid dizziness. Use a chair to stabilize yourself if necessary, and stop the exercise if dizziness becomes a problem. Hold each position of the head for 30 seconds before moving on to the next. Repeat two to three times.

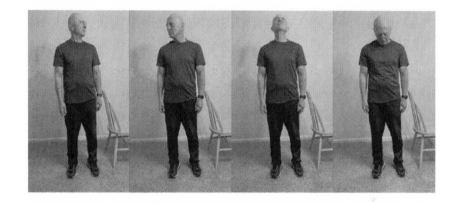

Clock Reach

While holding onto a chair with your left hand, gently lift the right foot only slightly off the ground and shift your weight to your left foot. Extend the right arm pointing out in front of you and hold for a moment. Then slowly move the arm pointing out to the side. After holding for another moment, try to point the arm behind you. It is okay if you're unable to point the arm behind yourself at first. Repeat on the other side. Repeat the whole sequence two to three times. With practice, flexibility will improve with this stretch. The Clock Reach helps with balance and core control of the body.

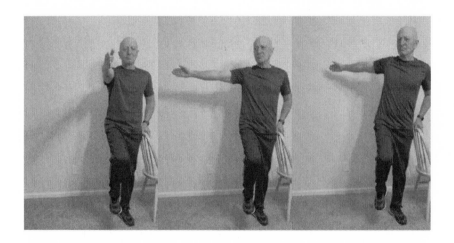

ALTERNATING VISION WALKS

To begin this exercise, stand at the end of a room with the feet placed shoulder-width apart. Turn the head to the left and take five steps while maintaining the head's position. Then stop, gently turn the head to the right, and take another five steps. Repeat this exercise five times with the head in each direction. This exercise will assist with balance and stability when in motion.

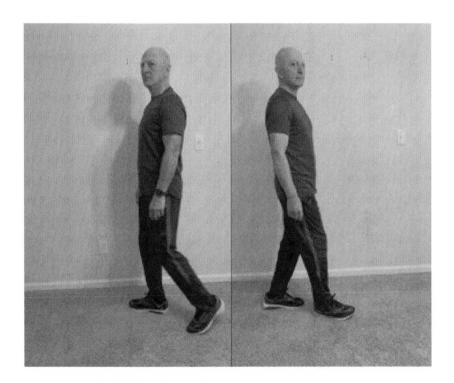

Body Circles

Body circles can be performed at a variety of levels of difficulty. Use a stabilizer if necessary to prevent becoming unbalanced. If a stabilizer is not needed, place your hands on your hips or out to the sides for added difficulty. Start the body circles by ensuring the lower portion of the body is supported and still with feet planted shoulder-width apart. Rotate the body in a circle ten times in each direction.

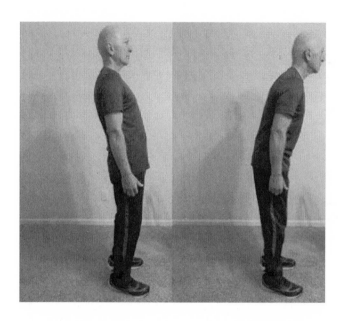

GRAPEVINE

This exercise is best enjoyed with some music to move to. Use your phone or stereo system to play a favorite song while making your way from one end of the room to the other and back again. Use a visual aid to move to your left in a straight line as follows. Shift your weight onto your left foot. Step left with your right foot moving around and in front of your left foot. Shift your weight onto the right foot. Then step left with your left foot moving behind and around your right foot. Finally, shift your weight back onto your left foot. Do this as you move to the left across the room, then switch legs, and move back to the other side of the room. Repeat two to three times.

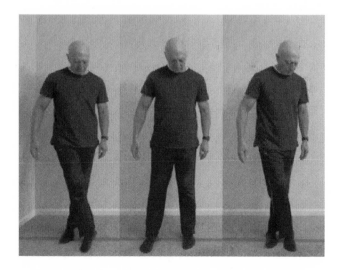

This dance can be made more difficult once you've gotten the hang of it, by looking out in front of yourself versus at the floor. If needed, use a long countertop or partner for support. The grapevine aids in coordination, balance, and strength training in the hips and legs.

Sit-To-Stands

This exercise is performed exactly as described, and can be aided by a stabilizer for better balance control. Stand close to the edge of a chair and sit down in a slow and controlled manner. Rest for a moment before standing again. Repeat the exercise ten times. Sit-to-stands mimic the everyday movement and can be responsible for a loss of balance at times. For added difficulty, you can perform this exercise while crossing your arms as shown below. Practicing regularly will assist with strengthening the muscles used to perform this movement.

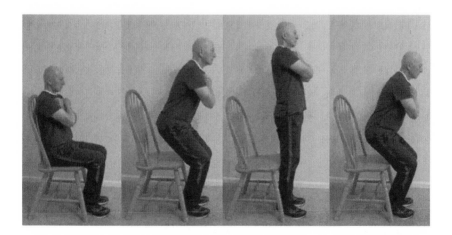

See videos of these exercises at www.betterbalanceforall.com

* * *

SAMPLE STANDING WEEKLY EXERCISE PLAN

Repeat these exercises over the next four weeks

Monday: Head Rotation, Single-Leg Stance, Narrow Stance Reaches, Standing Marches, Lateral Stepping

Tuesday: Head Rotation, Foot Taps to Step or Cone, Narrow Stance Reaches, Mini Lunges, Squats, Sit-to-Stands

Wednesday: Single-Leg Stance, Narrow Stance Reaches, Standing Marches, Lateral Stepping, Heel Raises

Thursday: Head Rotation, Foot Taps to Step or Cone, 3-Way Hip Kick, Mini Lunges, Grapevine

Friday: Head Rotation, Narrow Stance Reaches, Standing Marches, Alternating Vision Walks

Saturday: Single-Leg Stance, Lateral Stepping, Squats, Tandem or Semi-Tandem Stance

Sunday: Heel Raises, 3-Way Hip Kick, Lateral Stepping, Hamstring Stretch, Calf Stretch, Clock Reach, Body Circles

Strengthening muscles used in both the sitting and standing exercises is essential to improving coordination and overall balance. Getting into a routine of exercising will ensure that progress is made and will go a long way to restoring confidence in the ability to enjoy activities again. However, the most important muscles that need time and attention to restore optimum balance are the core muscles.

The next chapter will guide you on how to make sure the core muscles are properly conditioned.

HELP OTHERS FIND THIS BOOK

Science has shown that when you do something nice for someone else, it gives you and the other person a good feeling. This is the easiest way that kindness to strangers pays off. I would like to give you an opportunity to perform an act of kindness during your reading (or listening) experience.

People judge a book by the number of good reviews it has received. The only way for this book to reach many other readers who need it is to have as many reviews as possible.

If you have found this book to be of value so far, would you please take a moment right now and leave an honest review of this book and its contents? It will cost you nothing but it will help one more person who needs this book, find it and use its content to have a healthier and more active life.

This will take you less than a minute of your time. All you have to do is to leave a review.

This will also help this first-time writer.

If you are reading on kindle or an e-reader: Scroll to the bottom of the book, then swipe up and it will prompt a review.

If you are reading a print copy or none of the above work, please go to the page on Amazon (or where you purchased this book) and leave a review.

Thank you for your kindness.

Now, let's get back to the rest of this book.

4

CORE EXERCISES

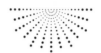

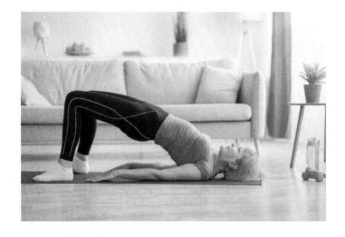

The core muscles consist of the back, abdominal, hip, and pelvic muscle groups. They work together to stabilize the limbs and spine for all of the body's movements. This makes the core muscles the most important muscle group for maintaining balance and stability. It may seem as though the exercises focused on in this book so far have included the entire body. And, although the core has been involved, we have yet to focus on strengthening it directly.

While the entire body contributes to balance and stability, the core muscles hold far more responsibility for maintaining our balance than we realize. So, it's time that some additional focus is taken to ensure they are strong and fit enough to provide the stable framework needed for everyday activities.

FIVE BENEFITS OF A STRONG CORE

One: A stronger core means better stability and balance.

Two: Having better balance and stability results in a reduced risk of falls and injuries.

Three: In addition to these benefits, they also allow for the rest of our body to become stronger by providing a sound framework to move from.

Four: A strong core reduces pain in the lower back from occurring.

Five: Improving strength in the core results in making tasks easier to accomplish.

With these benefits in mind, core exercises are essential to include in any exercise routine. They lay the groundwork for the ease and efficiency of all of the other exercises mentioned thus far. So without further ado, let's get started!

EXERCISES

Knees-To-Chest

Utilize a stable chair for this exercise and begin by sitting comfortably toward the front of the chair. Lean the shoulders back until they rest on the upper portion of the chair and grip the seat with both hands to brace and balance yourself. Start the exercise with both legs straight out in front of you with the heels resting on the ground. Then begin bending the knees as closely toward your chest as possible. Return the legs outstretched and resting with the heels on the ground. Repeat this motion of bringing the knees close to the chest 8 to 12 times to equal one set. Complete two to three sets. If unable to bring both knees toward the chest, modify the exercise by planting one foot on the ground firmly while raising one knee toward the chest.

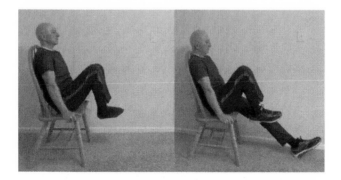

Extended Leg Raises

Also making use of a stable chair, begin by sitting toward the front of the seat. Engage the core and keep the back straight throughout this exercise. Grip the seat of the chair with both hands and place feet out in front of the body, heels gently resting on the ground, and with straight legs. Begin by lifting one leg in the air as high as possible and returning it to the ground in a controlled and gentle movement. Repeat this with the opposite leg to equal a single rep. Complete 8–12 reps for two to three total sets.

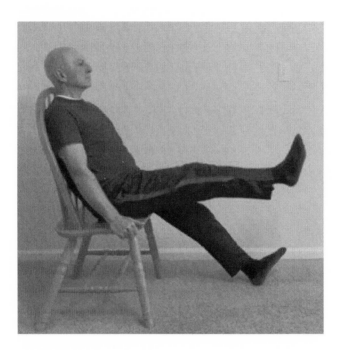

Leg Kicks

Again, while sitting toward the front of a stable chair, grip the seat and lean back in the chair for stability. Lift both feet, with legs straight, off of the ground with the intent of bringing them parallel to the hips. Begin slowly kicking one leg at a time, and in alteration with the other, a few inches higher into the air. Try to prevent the legs from resting on the ground during a set if possible. Kick alternating feet 8–12 times for a single set and complete two to three sets total.

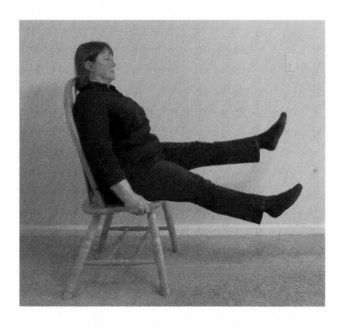

MODIFIED PLANKS

Stand facing a chair with a straight back. Grip the seat of the chair with both hands while keeping the elbows slightly bent. Step the feet backward a few feet until the shoulders align with the hands gripping the chair. It is important to keep the hips at a level position with the body and the tummy tucked inward. The back is to remain flat so that the body is fully aligned from shoulders to feet. Hold this position for 30 seconds and then stand or sit down for a short break. Repeat this exercise two to three times.

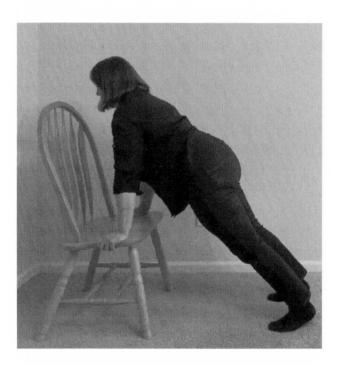

Tummy Twists

This exercise uses a medicine ball, a small weight, or an object that is a comfortable weight for lifting. Begin this exercise in a chair with both feet planted firmly on the ground. Lift the weight off of the lap and then twist slowly to the right while holding the weight at the center of the torso. Then rotate to the left for the completion of one rep. Perform eight to ten reps per set, two to three times, while taking short breaks between sets.

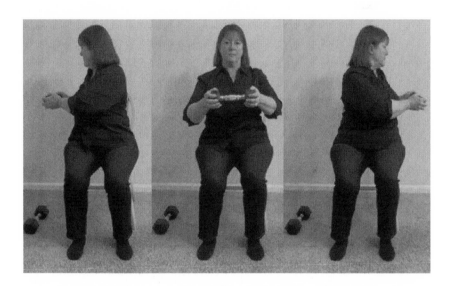

Side Bends

Sit upright in a stable chair with one hand placed behind the head, and the other stretched out to the side with a straight arm. While engaging the core muscles, bend the torso in the direction of the outstretched hand while reaching that hand toward the ground. Focus on using the muscles running along the rib cage when bending. Return to the upright position and repeat the exercise another 8–12 times before switching the bend to the opposite side. Perform two to three sets on each side.

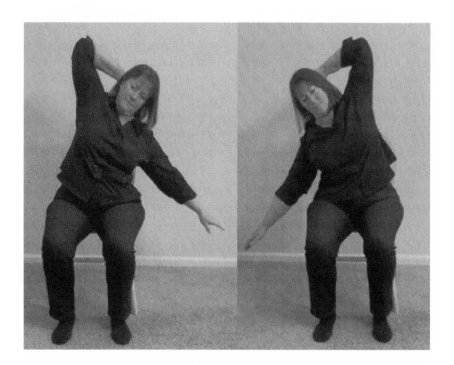

Leg Lifts

While seated toward the front of a stable chair, grip the seat with both hands, and lift one leg off the ground about four to five inches. Keep the knee straight and the core muscles engaged. Return the foot to the floor and then switch legs to perform the exercise on the opposite leg. Repeat this exercise eight to ten times on each leg to total one set. Perform two to three sets.

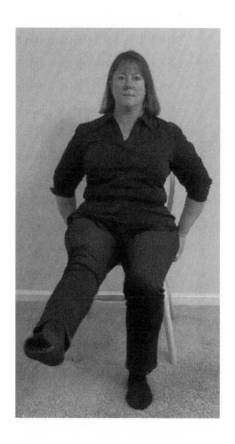

THE SUPERMAN

This exercise is performed while lying face-down on the ground with arms straight overhead and legs shoulder-width apart. Begin by lifting the head, right arm, and left leg a couple of inches off of the floor. Hold this position for two to three seconds before slowly returning to a resting position on the ground. Switch the arms and legs used for each rep. Perform eight to ten reps on each side for a total of two to three sets.

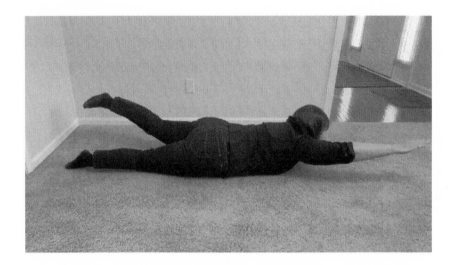

Wood Chops

Begin this exercise from a standing position, knees slightly bent, and feet a bit wider than shoulder-width apart. With the hands grasped together, bring the arms up over the right shoulder. While performing a slow squat, bring the hands down in a diagonal motion across the body and toward the left foot. Raise out of the squat slowly while bringing the hands back up and across above the shoulder again. Repeat the wood chop eight to ten times on each side for a total of two to three sets.

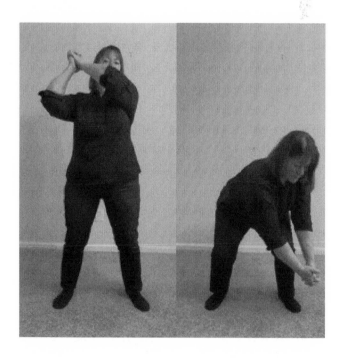

THE BRIDGE

Start the bridge by lying on the floor with bent knees and feet planted firmly on the ground. With a straight back, lift the hips from the ground while maintaining a tight core. Hold the hips up with an aligned body for a few seconds before slowly lowering the hips back to the floor. Repeat this exercise eight to ten times and take breaks as needed.

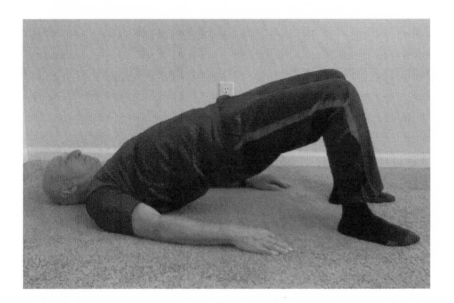

Modified Leg Lifts

Sit upright towards the front of a chair with the shoulders rolled back and the seat gripped with both hands. Begin with the knees and feet together while raising them slowly off of the ground a few inches. Hold them above the ground a moment before returning them to the floor in a controlled motion. Repeat this exercise 10–12 times per set for a total of three to five sets. If it feels too much to do this with both legs at the same time, just do one leg at a time as you see here.

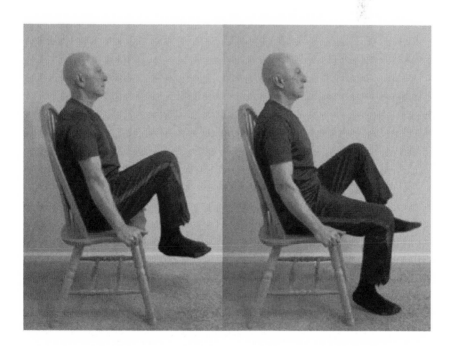

See videos of these exercises at www.betterbalanceforall.com

* * *

SAMPLE CORE EXERCISE PLAN

Monday: Extended Leg Raises, Leg Kicks, Tummy Twists, The Superman

Tuesday: Modified Planks, Wood Chops, Modified, Leg Lifts

Wednesday: Extended Leg Raises, The Superman, The Bridge

Thursday: Modified Planks, Knees-to-chest, Tummy Twists, Wood Chops

Friday: Extended Leg Raises, Leg Kicks, Knees-to-chest, Leg Lifts

Saturday: Modified Planks, Side Bends, Leg Lifts

Sunday: Side Bends, The Bridge

These core exercises will increase the body's capability to perform daily activities and contribute to a more confident sense of balance. After completing the exercises laid out so far, it is important to maintain flexible and relaxed muscles.

The next chapter covers stretches that will help relieve muscle tension in several areas of the body.

5

STRETCHING EXERCISES

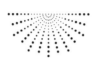

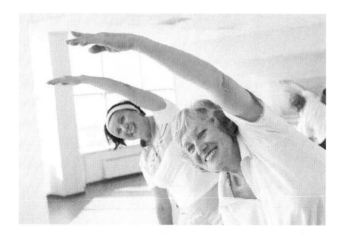

P erforming these exercises and stretches improves one's physical fitness, but it is essential to also maintain a positive mental state as well. It can be incredibly stressful to go through the golden years of your life being scared of falling. And, while the exercises in this book will boost your confidence, stretching has profound benefits that contribute to a stronger and more assured mind and body, as well.

BENEFITS OF STRETCHING

The five major benefits of stretching include: an **improved range of movement, better posture, less tension and soreness in the muscles, reduced risk of injury, increased circulation,** and **better muscle control**. Stretching improves balance and coordination. It prepares the body for movement by loosening the muscles and distributing oxygen and nutrients to the tissues. Stretching exercises also slow down joint degeneration by preventing muscle stiffness and aiding in recovery after an accident or injury. They support proper posture by increasing flexibility and supporting the lower back and shoulders, as well as providing a power boost to the brain from the increased blood flow.

TYPES OF STRETCHING

There are two primary types of stretching covered in this section. These are **dynamic and static stretching. Dynamic stretching** involves movements that are done repeatedly over a short period. They assist with warming up and loosening the muscles and are ideal to perform before physical activity. Another common technique is called **static stretching,** which involves movements that elongate the muscle while loosening it, and are held for a considerably longer time. Typically, dynamic stretches are held for about eight to ten seconds while static stretches are held for about 15–30 seconds. Static stretches provide increased blood flow to the muscles and are ideal for after workouts to prevent soreness. They also aid in muscle recovery after exercise or an injury.

FOCUS POINTS WHILE STRETCHING

Warming up and cooling down should be incorporated into the stretching routine. By getting the heart pumping beforehand, the muscles will respond to the stretch more readily. Also, a quick walk after stretching will maximize the benefits of the stretch. While stretching, remind yourself to breathe consistently and comfortably. Be conscious of the stretch and always perform them with ease. Stretching can sometimes reveal stiffness and be uncomfortable, but it should never be painful.

Speak to your physician before starting any exercise or stretching program and discuss any conditions that may present a hazard. And, if at any point you begin experiencing pain, talk to a physician immediately.

If the pain does present itself, stop the exercise or stretch right away. Continuously take even breaths so that oxygen is flowing at all times. Avoid bouncing into a stretch to prevent any injuries from occurring. All stretches should be done in

an easy and gentle motion. Keep the back in proper alignment whenever turning so as not to pinch a nerve. And
lastly, avoid overextending the head backward. With the
spinal column running at the base of the neck, bending it too
far backward can lead to serious injury, pain, or dizziness.

STATIC STRETCHES

You might be asking what it is about static stretching that
promotes the feeling of relaxation and greater flexibility
(often the biggest sign of muscle recovery post-exercise). It is
common knowledge that there are benefits to stretching, but
what makes static stretching unique? And, why is it of particular importance after exercising? There are distinct beneficial elements of static stretching that we'll discuss now,
beginning with blood flow.

Blood Flow: Static stretching has an interesting effect on the
blood flow to a muscle. During the stretch, the muscle is
elongated which contracts blood vessels and reduces the
flow of blood and nutrients to the muscle for the duration of
the stretch. When the stretch is over, and the muscle returns
to its' natural state, blood surges into the muscle. The blood
flow level is significantly greater after the stretch than before
the stretch began. This results in a mass-delivery of nutrients
as well as improved removal of cell metabolic waste. The
effect that static stretching has on blood flow is a direct
contributor to the muscle's recovery.

Relaxation: Static stretching directly induces the parasympathetic nervous system for up to weeks after the stretch is completed. This is the system that is responsible for feeling relaxed. A study found that when static stretching was completed for 15 minutes a day for 28 days, lasting effects were seen as improved changes in heart performance. (Walker, 2016)

Flexibility: Static stretching improves the range of motion of a joint and thus increases the flexibility of that joint. Increasing flexibility and having greater range of motion enables the muscles to work and perform a variety of motions that would otherwise be inhibited.

ARM RAISES

Stand with the feet a comfortable distance apart and the hands relaxed down at your sides. Roll the shoulders back and lift the chest to the sky for proper posture. Reach the arms straight up over your head with a slow and deep inhale and hold for six or seven seconds. Slowly relax the arms back down to your sides while exhaling and repeat three or four times.

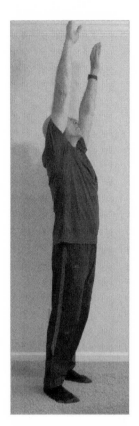

HANDS AND WRISTS

Reach your arms out in front of you with the palms facing downwards. Stretch the fingers out and rotate the wrists. This can also be done with the arms down and at your sides. Repeat this ten times or for one minute.

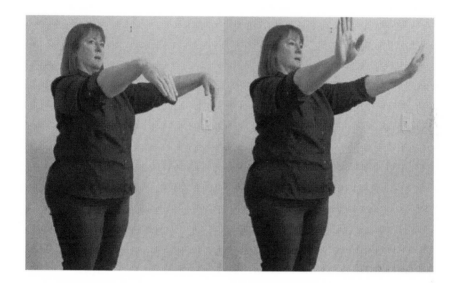

CHEST

While comfortably seated, bring the arms up with bent elbows and rest your hands gently at the back of your head. Inhale and bring the upper torso back as far as possible to feel a stretch across the chest. Repeat this three or four times.

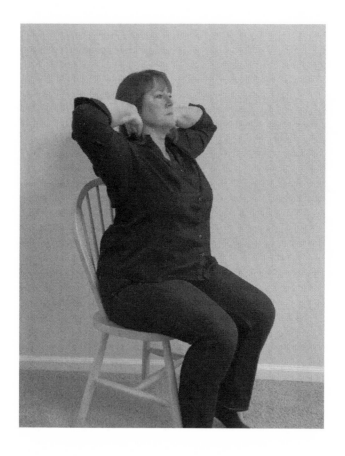

UPPER BACK

Standing up straight, reach your hands behind you with fingers intertwined. Take a breath in, and when exhaling, lift your arms behind you a bit further, slightly bending forward. Hold the pose for a 10 seconds before returning your arms to your sides in a comfortable position. Repeat this stretch ten times.

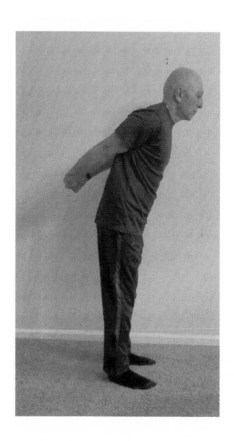

LOWER BACK

While standing up straight, brace your hands' palms down on your bottom. Push the ribcage out front while leaning the shoulders slightly backward to feel a stretch in the lower back. Hold for 10 seconds before returning the torso to a neutral position. Repeat this stretch seven times.

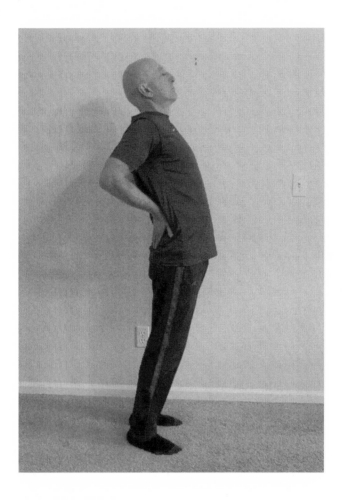

HAMSTRINGS

Sit down comfortably on the floor or a sturdy bench with one leg fully extended out in front and the other bent with the foot slightly inward toward the body. Slowly reach out toward the extended leg as far as possible. Start with reaching for the knee for a few moments and then to your foot. Hold the stretch for about 25 seconds before coming up to a neutral position. Repeat this stretch on the opposite leg.

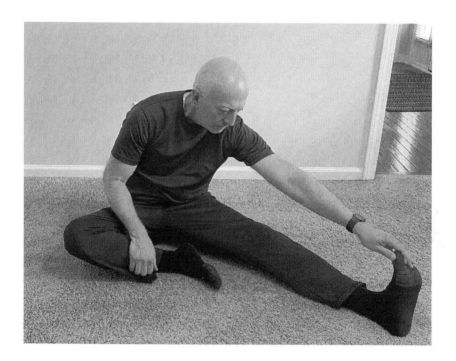

QUADRICEPS

Using a chair for balance and support, bend one knee and reach behind to grasp the ankle for 20 seconds. Gently release the ankle and repeat the stretch on the opposite leg.

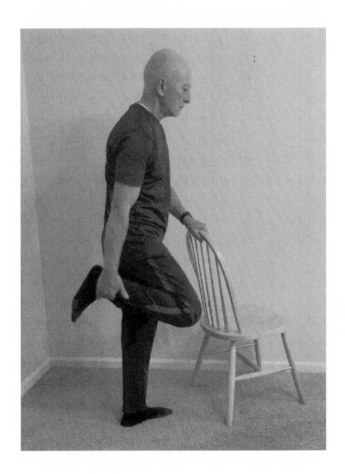

KNEES

While seated, bend the right knee upwards and gently pull it towards your chest. Take a breath and stretch the knee for ten seconds, before slowly returning the foot to the ground. Repeat on the opposite knee. If you are experiencing difficulty, you can use your hands to bring your knee up.

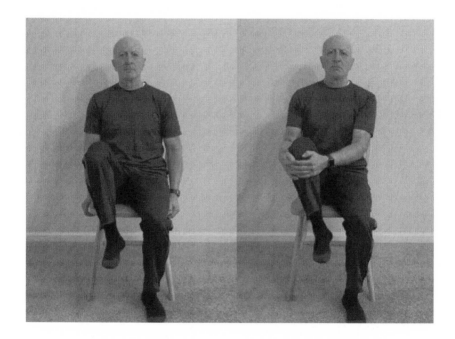

CALVES

Using a countertop or wall for support, use both hands to brace yourself while stepping one foot toward the wall. With both feet flat on the floor, bring your hips toward the wall and hold for 30 seconds. Repeat and stretch the opposite calf.

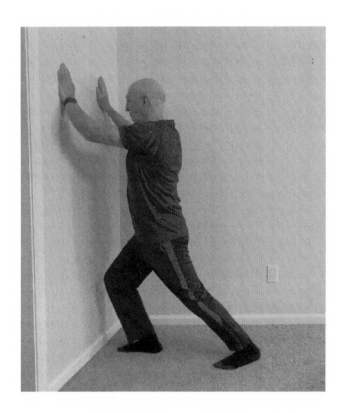

ANKLES

While sitting, bring one leg up and rest it on the opposite knee. Rotate the ankle slowly 10–12 times one way and then repeat in the opposite direction. Do this for each ankle.

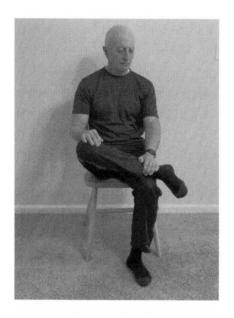

DYNAMIC STRETCHES

Dynamic stretches are slow and controlled movements that take a joint to its limit of mobility. They benefit the muscle by preparing it for movement which results in a reduced risk of injury during the exercise. Ideally, one should perform movements like those they are about to do in the exercise. The primary benefit of dynamic stretching for senior citizens is that they improve the joint's range of motion thus increasing one's mobility.

Imagine not having the limitations of stiff shoulders or hips anymore. Tripping over a rug or squeezing through a tight space wouldn't seem so scary. Having the confidence to know that you would easily catch yourself or be able to maneuver close quarters can make all the difference in the activities we choose to do. Dynamic stretches should be performed for about 10 to 15 minutes before an exercise.

NECK TURNS

While sitting comfortably in a chair and resting your feet flat on the ground, rotate the head slowly to one side. Hold the stretch for about 20–30 seconds before returning it to the forward-facing neutral position. Repeat this stretch three to five times in each direction.

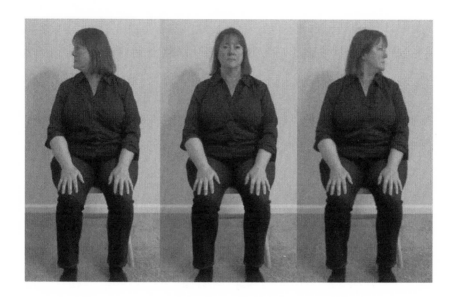

Seated Backbend

Perform this stretch while sitting in a stable chair toward the front of the seat. With both feet planted on the ground, hands braced on the knees, bend the upper back backward until a stretch is felt but is not painful. Hold this pose for about 20 seconds before returning to the neutral upright position. Repeat the exercise three to five times.

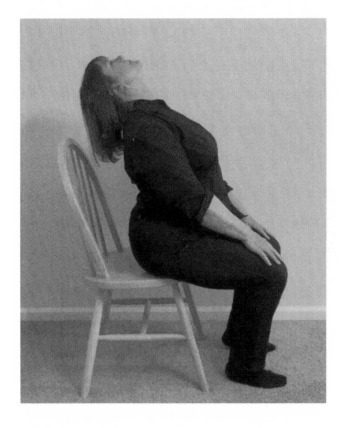

Seated Overhead Stretch

While sitting at the edge of a stable chair, place feet flat on the floor, and raise the hands straight into the air with the fingers intertwined. Slowly arch backward and push the stomach out to feel a stretch in the abdomen. Hold the pose for about 20 seconds before lowering the hands and returning to the neutral seated position. Repeat the stretch three to five times.

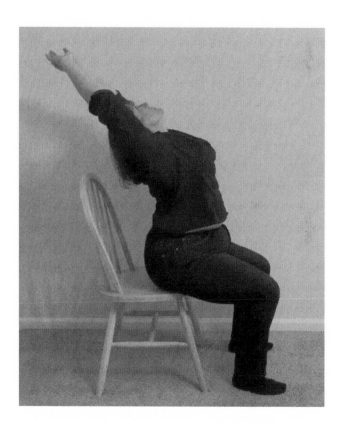

SEATED SIDE STRETCH

Begin this stretch sitting comfortably in a chair towards the front of the seat with the feet planted on the ground. While gripping the seat of the chair with one hand, raise the other hand overhead and bend to the opposite side. This should create a stretching feeling along the side of the body with the hand raised in the air. Be sure to keep the shoulders square in this stretch to get its maximum benefit. Hold the position for about 20 seconds before switching to the other side. Repeat the stretch three to five times on each side.

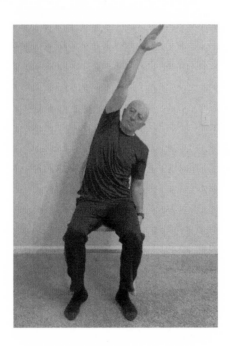

Seated Hip Stretch

Sitting at the edge of a chair in a comfortable and stable position, raise one leg and rest it at the ankle on top of the knee of the opposite leg. Hold this position for about 20 seconds to feel a stretch in the hips. For an additional stretch, lean the body forward until a stretch is felt. Perform this stretch on each leg two to three times.

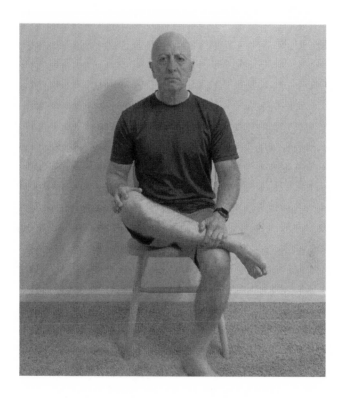

Hip Circles

Using stationary support, such as a wall or countertop, brace yourself while lifting one leg out to the side with a straight knee. Rotate the leg in slow and controlled circles. Complete 20 circles in each direction and then repeat on the opposite leg.

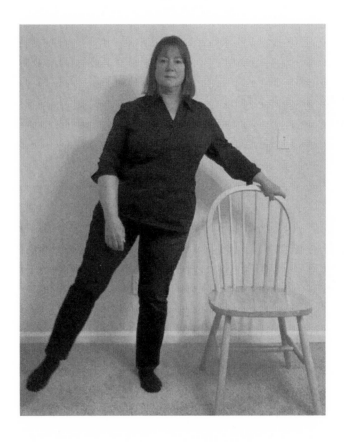

ARM CIRCLES

Sitting or standing, hold the arms out straight to the sides level to the shoulders. Circle the arms forwards 20 times and then backward another 20 times. For a deeper stretch, increase the size of the circles.

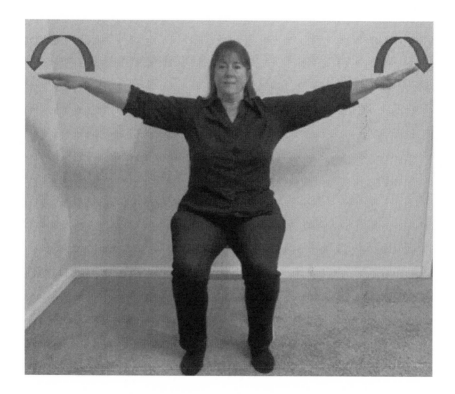

ARM SWINGS

Stand with both arms parallel to each other and out in front of the body. Begin walking while swinging the arms back and forth together from left, to right, to left, etc., using only the shoulders to create the motion in the arms. The head and torso should remain facing forward as you walk. Complete 30 seconds of arm swings.

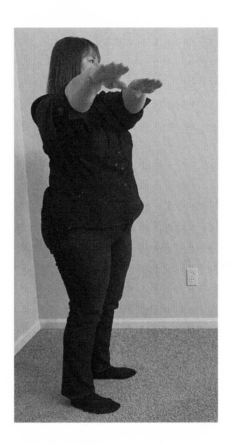

Heel-To-Toe Walk

This stretch helps with ankle mobility and warm up the shin and calf muscles. Start by moving one foot forward keeping the ankle flexed, the knee straight, then lean forward to feel a stretch in the calf and behind the leg. Roll forward onto the ball of your foot and come up into a heel raise on both feet. Then alternate legs and repeat five times.

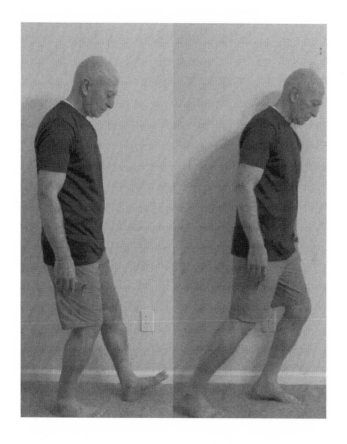

Lunges

Using a wall for support, begin with the feet placed shoulder-width apart and one hand braced on the wall. Step the right foot out as far as possible without losing balance. Then lower the left knee toward the ground. Be sure to keep the knee from going beyond the ankle and only drop the knee to a level that enables a stretch but does not produce pain. Perform this stretch five times on each leg.

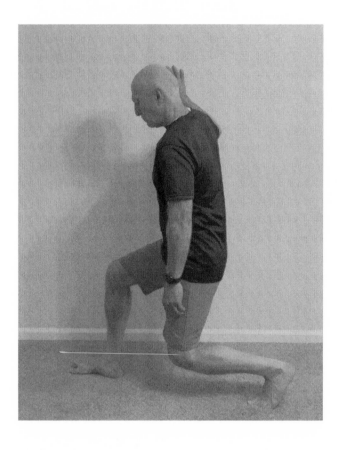

See videos of these exercises at www.betterbalanceforall.com

* * *

SAMPLE STRETCHING EXERCISE PLAN

We have listed both static and dynamic exercise days here. You can alternate static and dynamic exercise days.

Monday: Static Exercises: Hamstrings, Quadriceps, Knees, Calves, Ankles

Monday: Dynamic Exercises: Seated Hip Stretch, Hip Circles

Tuesday: Static Exercises: Chest, Upper Back, Lower Back

Tuesday: Dynamic Exercises: Neck Turns, Seated Back-bend, Seated Overhead Stretch, Seated Side Stretch

Wednesday: Static Exercises: Hamstrings, Quadriceps, Knees, Calves, Ankles

Wednesday: Dynamic Exercises: Seated Hip Stretch, Hip Circles

Thursday: Static Exercises: Chest, Upper Back, Lower Back

Thursday: Dynamic Exercises: Neck Turns, Seated Back-bend, Seated Overhead Stretch, Seated Side Stretch

Friday: Static Exercises: Arm Raises, Hands, and Wrists

Friday: Dynamic Exercises: Arm Circles, Arm Swings

Saturday: Static Exercises: Hamstrings, Quadriceps, Knees, Calves, Ankles

Saturday: Dynamic Exercises: Heal-to-Toe Walk, Lunges With a Twist

Sunday: Static Exercises: Arm Raises, Hands, and Wrists

Sunday: Dynamic Exercises: Heal-to-Toe Walk, Lunges With a Twist, Arm Circles, Arm Swings

STRETCHING SPORTS

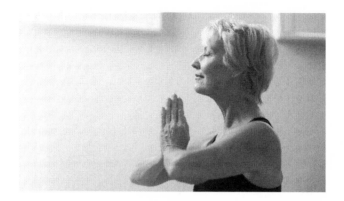

Several sports can be taken up at any age and provide exercise and stretching intrinsically. These sports teach new skills while also introducing you to a community of support and common interest.

Yoga

Yoga is a common choice for seniors and is wonderful for strengthening the body, relieving stress, stretching, improving sleep, and getting involved with a community of health-conscious people. Yoga provides a wonderful natural release of endorphins which can uplift our mood and be an additional source of energy throughout the day. If yoga is done consistently, it can also be a great way to increase bone density and is safe enough for those living with osteoporosis to perform.

If there isn't a yoga class offered where you live, find a senior citizens yoga YouTube video and practice a couple of days a week and invite your friends to join in on the fun. There are also community centers and private studios that can offer yoga classes with modified movements to fit your needs. If you find yoga to be especially enjoyable, look into senior citizens' yoga retreats. They can be extremely relaxing and give opportunities to make new acquaintances.

Pilates

Pilates is another sport that involves stretching, muscle strength, and breathing. Pilates results in improved strength, endurance, stability, and balance. The small movements can be modified so that anyone can participate and receive substantial benefits. Pilates focuses on small and specific exercises but also emphasizes breathing techniques that improve circulation and blood flow.

There is likely a pilates studio close by that you can join. They often offer walk-in classes, monthly memberships, and package deals. Pilates studios also tend to offer gift certificates so don't forget to mention to family and friends that you'd like to give it a try for your birthday.

Swimming

The last stretching sport that we'll mention here is swimming. Swimming is the perfect option for a low-impact sport that gently stretches, elongates, and strengthens the muscles. It also provides cardiovascular benefits for improved endurance and circulation. The motions used to swim are gentle enough to avoid straining the muscles and contribute to added flexibility.

The one downfall of swimming is that it obviously cannot be done just anywhere. The first step toward making swimming part of your regular exercise routine is identifying where the most convenient pool is located. Once that piece of the puzzle is solved, swimming will prove to be an extremely versatile sport. There are often classes that are taught just for senior citizens at local gyms or recreation centers such as your local YMCA, and those can be a lot of fun! But, if the most convenient pool to swim in happens to be in your backyard, you're in luck. Swimming laps or looking up particular water exercises are an easy way to go as well. Think about inviting the grandkids over to join you. They would likely have fun doing the exercises as well.

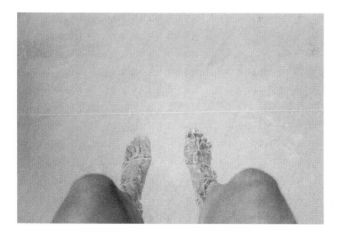

Exercising and stretching are critical to improving balance and stability because they build up our physical abilities and improve confidence in daily activities. However, there is more to staying balanced than being physically fit. Other factors are important to consider as well. In the next chapter, we'll explore another facet of maintaining stability and control.

6

IMPROVING BALANCE THROUGH INNER EAR AND VESTIBULAR EXERCISES

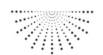

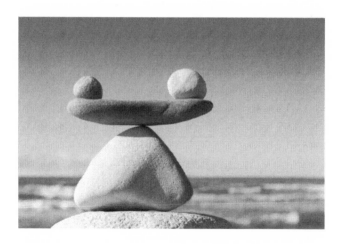

W e often don't think of the inner ear as a culprit of the loss of balance. However, because the inner ear deteriorates as we age, it often contributes to instability and shaky confidence when going about day-to-day activities. The inner ear can make us feel entirely in control of our physical stability, or it can cause us to feel as if we're on a small boat in a hurricane. There isn't a lot that can be done about aging, but there is plenty that we can do to strengthen the inner ear and restore confidence and control on our feet. The goal of this chapter is to show you what is possible.

BALANCE EXERCISES FOR THE INNER EAR

Before beginning the next series of exercises, it is important to consult a physician about possible vertigo-like symptoms you may be experiencing. They should be able to recommend which exercises could work best for you and any that you should possibly avoid. I strongly believe that these exercises should be done under the supervision of a trained practitioner. Thus, a description of these exercises is provided here to give you a better idea of what is involved. However, I do not provide pictures or videos of these exercises (although these can be easily found online), because we want you to avoid performing these exercises on your own.

The inner ear contains calcium crystals, which should all adhere to the inner ear walls. If a crystal detaches from the wall, it can cause serious balance issues and make a person feel as though they are spinning even when they're standing still. This sensation can be extremely disruptive, but there are several ways to go about treating this type of vertigo, also known as Benign Paroxysmal Positional Vertigo (BPPV). The exercises outlined here can assist with correcting the inner ear issue but should be strictly supported by the recommendation of a physician.

The Epley Maneuver

The Epley Maneuver is a series of head movements that are designed to coax a loose crystal to move from the position which is causing the vertigo symptoms.

Sit at the edge of a bed with a pillow placed behind you. Turn your head in the direction that you feel the vertigo is originating from and quickly lie back, allowing your back and shoulders to rest on the pillow, while your head is inclined slightly backward. Keep your head turned as you lie back and hold it in that direction while lying down for 30 seconds. Then, slightly turn the head in the opposite direction for 30 more seconds. Finally, turn the head the rest of the way in the same direction, wait another 30 seconds, and sit back up with the head still turned. Repeat this process three times a day until the vertigo symptoms stop for 24 hours.

The Semont Maneuver

The Semont Maneuver is only recommended if the Epley Maneuver did not correct the vertigo symptoms. Consult a physician before attempting the maneuver to discuss any physical limitations to avoid injury.

Begin this maneuver by sitting at the edge of a bed with the head turned away from where vertigo seems to be originating from. Then lie down quickly on the opposite side of the body while keeping the head turned. Stay in this position for about two to three minutes. Next, flip over and lie on the other side while still keeping the head turned and remaining for 30 seconds before sitting up slowly. Repeat this series of motions three times until vertigo symptoms have been relieved for 24 hours.

The Foster Maneuver

While the Foster Maneuver does not address correcting the position of crystals within the inner ear, it can provide relief from vertigo and improve balance. It is also referred to as a "half somersault".

Begin the Foster Maneuver by kneeling on the floor and sitting back on the heels of your feet. Bend the head back to look up at the ceiling for 30 seconds. Then quickly bring your chin to your chest and bend your body at the waist to bring your head down to the ground between your knees. Wait here another 30 seconds. Now turn your head in the direction of the affected ear and remain in this position for 30 more seconds. Then bring your upper body up, with the head still turned, and brace the hands on the floor with the head in line with the body for 30 seconds. Lastly, look up toward the ceiling again, still with the head turned, and stand up slowly. It is recommended that a few repetitions are done in a single day to rectify the vertigo symptoms.

The Brandt-Daroff Exercise

The Brandt-Daroff Exercise is a quick and easy variation of the Foster maneuver, and should be performed at least twice a day until there are no remaining symptoms of vertigo. Begin the exercise sitting at the edge of a bed. Tilt the head at a 45-degree angle and lie down quickly to one side. When the vertigo symptom passes, sit up slowly and repeat the exercise on the opposite side.

Vestibular Rehabilitation

There are two main types of exercises that are used during vestibular rehabilitation, known as **habituation exercises** and **gaze stabilization exercises**. Both are performed with the supervision and direction of a licensed physician.

Do not try these exercises at home.

The habituation exercises involve triggering the particular actions that cause a person to feel vertigo while in a safe surrounding of soft surfaces. The idea is that this will condition the brain to stabilize the vertigo feeling by building up a tolerance to the stimulation. Over time, the person will adjust to the trigger quickly and not feel the symptoms of vertigo anymore.

The gaze stabilization exercises involve the person suffering from vertigo staring at a fixed object while turning and moving their head. The exercise aims to heal damage in the inner ear by using vision and somatosensation stimulation.

THE INNERWORKINGS OF VESTIBULAR EXERCISES

The goals of vestibular exercises are to retrain the brain to interpret the motion of the eyes and head as independent of one another and produce a stabilization effect. Using these exercises, one should practice the head motions that make them dizzy and build up a tolerance to the stimulation. This is done by practicing similar movements to those used in everyday life to develop a sense of awareness by the eyes and muscles. The exercises aim to increase comfort and confidence with movements both in daylight and in darkness. They assist in building up movement confidence to induce effortless and spontaneous movements that do not result in loss of balance and stability.

Before beginning these exercises, be sure to consult a physician to discuss any potential limitations or modifications that should be considered. Also, in the beginning, it is recommended to have a support person present that can step in and assist if necessary. Vocalize what you are feeling to them during the exercise so that they can call for help if the dizziness becomes too much.

The vestibular exercise program should be performed over 6 to 12 weeks. It is okay to stop the exercises at any point if the dizziness entirely resolves. Keep in mind that if the exercises are not continued while vertigo persists, the symptoms could become worse. Be sure that the vertigo is entirely resolved by continuing the exercises for two full weeks symptom-free. The exercises can always be started again should dizzy symptoms return. Note that these exercises are designed to induce the feeling of dizziness and should not be stopped unless one is unable to proceed. At that point, a physician or nurse should be consulted.

Retraining the brain is hard and uncomfortable work, but persistence will pay off with increased balance and confidence in your movements. Let's get started!

VESTIBULAR EXERCISES

As with other exercise programs, starting this new exercise routine may be difficult at first. Be understanding with yourself and do your best. It may take time, but eventually, each exercise should be performed in sets of 20 repetitions. Start slowly and build up speed as you are able. Know that you will likely become dizzy, and that it is important to continue. Stop for a moment and take deep breaths if you feel yourself becoming nauseous. If you need to, move on to a different exercise and come back to the one that made you ill at the next session. We'll begin with the head exercises.

Head Exercises

For the head bending exercise, tilt the head to the ceiling and then to the floor, and precede this motion by using the eyes to focus on each appropriately. Do this for ten repetitions, break for 30 seconds, and repeat for two more sets of ten.

For the head-turning exercise, begin in a seated position. Turn the head to the left and then to the right, all while leading the movement with the eyes focused in the direction the head is turning. Pretend you're watching a ball bounce from one side of the room to the other. The motion should be done quickly enough to make you a bit dizzy but not so fast as to injure your neck. Repeat the motion ten times, break for 30 seconds, and complete two additional sets of ten in the same manner.

Modify this exercise as it becomes easier to include closed eyes and eventually standing while performing the head bends and turns. When standing is eventually incorporated, start with the feet about shoulder-width apart and then move them closer together as the exercise becomes easier.

Sitting

Perform each exercise a total of 20 times.

Shoulder Shrug: While sitting, shrug the shoulders up and down.

Head Turn: Turn the shoulders to the left and then to the right.

Torso Turn: Rotate the entire upper torso and head to the left with the eyes open, and then again with the eyes closed. Repeat the torso turn on the right in the same manner.

Forward Bend: Bend all the way forward, touching the floor if possible, and sit back up while keeping the gaze focused on a wall in front of you.

Forward Bend with Eye Movement: Repeat the last motion, but with the eyes following a gaze to the floor and back as well.

Up and Down Eye Movements: Keeping the head still, move the eyes up and down.

Side-to-Side Eye Movements: Move the eyes right to left and back.

Finger Focus: Bring your finger to the tip of your nose and back out again all while keeping the focus on the finger.

Standing

Sit and Stand: Begin in a seated position, raise to standing, and then sit back down again. Repeat this exercise 20 times.

Eyes Closed Sit and Stand: Do the sit-to-stand exercise again but with the eyes closed. Repeat it, but with the eyes closed, another 20 times.

Standing Balance: Stand facing into a corner of a room with one foot aligned with, and close to, the other foot. As this exercise becomes easier, decrease any gap between the toe of one foot and the heel of the other. Stand this way for 30 seconds. For an added challenge, do this exercise with your eyes closed without having to reach out for the wall.

Standing Balance with a Pillow: Again, standing into a corner of the room, stand on top of some pillows or cushions and try not to reach out to the wall for balance. Hold the pose for 30 seconds. The closer the feet are together, the more difficult this exercise becomes.

Basic Ball Throw: Throw a ball from one hand to the other above eye level 20 times.

Complex Ball Throw: Throw a ball from one hand to the other underneath one knee 20 times.

Heel-to-Heel Standing Balance: Stand with the heels of your feet together while staring straight ahead for 30 seconds. Have a friend stand close by for this exercise.

One Foot Standing Balance: Also with assistance, stand on one foot for 30 seconds. When this exercise becomes easier, repeat it with your eyes closed.

Various Balance Activities: Complete an array of other activities that can compromise balance such as stretching, climbing stairs, bending over or stooping, etc. Engage assistance as needed.

Walking

Heel-to-Toe Walk: Walk from heel to toe, in a straight line, from one end of a room to the other. Try to leave no gap between the toe of the first foot and the heel of the second. Walk like this for approximately five minutes. Use a nearby wall, or a partner, for support if necessary.

Heel-to-Toe Walk with Eye Movement: For a length of about 20 feet, walk while moving the head and eyes from left to right when the right foot steps forward, and then right to left when the left foot steps forward. Repeat the length of 20 feet walking like this three times. Then, for another three lengths, walk while moving the head and eyes up and down with each step. Perform this walking exercise another three lengths of 20 feet.

Lying Down

Begin by sitting at the edge of a bed. Lie down and swing the legs and feet up to rest on the bed. Complete this in one quick and fluid motion and then rest on the bed for 30 seconds, before sitting up and repeating the action three more times.

Eye Exercises

Before starting the eye exercises, there are a few things to take note of. The goal of the exercise is for the target to stay in focus and not become blurry or appear as though it is moving when the head is not. Only move the head slightly; about 45 degrees to each side. Move the head as quickly as possible while keeping the object in focus.

Be sure to utilize necessary prescription eyewear while performing these exercises. If you become dizzy or nauseous, try to push through the exercise. If you need to, take a short break and deep breaths to stabilize the vision again. Be sure to rest between the exercises and avoid any distractions. Turning the phone on silent and working in a quiet space will help.

And, just to be safe, be sure to work within reach of a wall or partner that you can reach out to in case of loss of balance. Let's begin.

Gaze Stabilization: Using an object to keep in focus between three and ten feet away, move the head left and right for 30 seconds. Continuing to keep the object in focus, move the head up and down for another 30 seconds. Keep in mind that having a busy printed background can make keeping the object in focus more difficult. Begin this exercise at your most comfortable level of difficulty and move up in difficulty as you're able. You may begin by first sitting in a chair, then move to a standing position with feet wider apart. Eventually, move the feet closer together and work toward marching in place while keeping focus and balance.

Smooth Pursuit: While keeping an object in focus, move it side to side while following it with the eyes and keeping the head still. Proceed for 30 seconds and then rest. Work toward performing this exercise while standing for a total of 20 times.

Varied Pursuit: While holding an object to keep in focus, move the object along with your head and eyes in an up and down motion for 30 seconds. Begin in a seated position and work up in difficulty to a standing position as you're able.

Opposing Pursuit: Hold an object out in front of you and keep it in focus while moving it up and down, then left and right. Move the head in the opposite direction of the object but do not lose focus. This exercise can be performed from a seated position, and eventually from a standing position for increased difficulty.

Romberg Exercise

Stand with the feet placed as closely together as possible and arms down at your sides. Be sure to ask for the assistance of a support person or stand near stabilizing props, such as a chair or wall, in case you lose your balance. Hold this stance while looking straight ahead for about 30 seconds.

Standing Sway

The standing sway should be done twice a day for about 30 seconds at a time. In the beginning, do this exercise while looking out in front of you and work up to doing it with your eyes closed. Be sure to have a chair to hold on to nearby if you get dizzy. With the feet shoulder-width apart, begin by shifting the body's weight from the right to the left and back again. Sway the body slowly and keep the feet firmly planted on the ground. Do this 30 times to each side. Then sway forwards and backward while continuing to keep the feet planted. Shift your weight onto your toes without lifting the heels of the foot off of the floor. Then shift your weight back onto your heels. Perform the standing sway forwards and backward 30 times as well.

Marching in Place

While standing near a corner of a room, perform a standing march lifting the knees high into the air 20 to 30 times. Use the wall to balance if you begin to fall. Try to repeat this exercise three times per day and aim toward performing it with your eyes closed.

Turning in Place

With a chair or wall nearby to grab for support if needed, turn the body in a half-circle. Try to turn quickly to the right, pause for ten seconds, then turn quickly to the left. Focus on practicing turning in the direction that makes you dizzier. Perform five turns three times per day.

Final Note: Deterioration of the inner ear is a product of aging that we cannot avoid altogether, but we can work to remedy the symptoms of it by performing these exercises. It is recommended that any condition that could be contributing to instability be fully investigated by a physician. And, while the inner ear may be giving you trouble, don't forget to get involved with physical exercise as well. The exercises mentioned in this chapter can be performed in addition to those in previous chapters for a fully-rounded fitness program that is sure to have you stable and in control again in just 28 days.

To continue down the path of discovering anything that could be leading to a fear of falling, the next chapter will address another common ailment of aging, arthritis.

Arthritis can make exercising seem impossible. However, not only is it possible, but it's necessary, regardless of age. It can be modified to meet the needs of those experiencing pain and discomfort while still offering muscle strengthening benefits. Read on to the next chapter for modified exercises to avoid arthritic pain.

7

SAFE EXERCISES TO DO IF YOU
HAVE ARTHRITIS

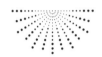

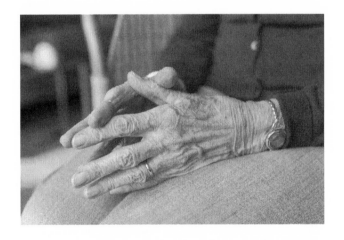

rthritis pain does not have to keep you from exercising to regain your sense of balance and control. There is a misconception that exercising will inflame arthritis, and therefore should be avoided. Thankfully, there is an array of exercises that can be done even if you have arthritis. They can be performed with the confidence that balance will improve without any unnecessary pain. There is no need to avoid exercising and gaining the stability and control that everyone deserves. Follow the exercises outlined here to work toward better balance while keeping arthritic pain at bay.

Having arthritis should be considered another reason to work toward better balance and stability because arthritic pain can alter the way we move. Walking may become difficult due to arthritic pain, falls become more of a risk, and injuries weaken the muscles. It's a vicious cycle—and the only way to break the cycle is by working to strengthen the muscles and avoid injuries by improving stability. Tai Chi, pool exercises, balancing exercises, walking, weight training, yoga, and stretching are all low-impact exercises that contribute to strength, agility, and endurance, which will greatly improve balance and stability.

Some things should be considered before you begin exercising if you have arthritis.

First and foremost, talk with your doctor about your condition and intentions of the exercises you'd like to try. They can advise the best way to go about them and suggest any necessary modifications. They may also suggest that a physical therapist is consulted about the exercises. Seeking professional advice will increase your confidence in starting a new exercise program.

Also, don't forget to warm-up before beginning the exercises to prevent any pulled muscles or other injuries. Check the equipment you'll be using to be sure it is in good working order. Be sure there is sufficient space clear of tripping hazards. Wear appropriate clothing that will allow freedom of movement. Start with a partner or assistant that can help guide the movements.

Lastly, be sure to stop immediately if you experience pain and consult a physician. New workout routines can be uncomfortable but they shouldn't ever be painful.

EXERCISES

Tai Chi

Tai Chi was developed in China as a martial art that consists of slow and fluid movements. The focus of Tai Chi is balance and control, so it is perfect as a fall prevention exercise. It reduces the weakness of the muscles and pain in the joints. It also improves flexibility. The low-impact movements are gentle enough that they can be performed by anyone with any type of arthritis without inducing a painful flare-up. While it is often offered at studios for private lessons, we've provided a full weekly routine that you can manage on your own or with a friend. Take a look at chapter eight for details of specific Tai Chi movements and their benefits.

Pool Exercises

Pool exercises make use of resistance in the water to exercise muscles without any painful impact or risk of falling. A warm water pool can ease aches and pains while providing a safe atmosphere for weight loss, stability, and endurance improvement exercises. Water exercise classes are a great way to begin and stick with a new exercise program. They provide guidance, support, and a wonderful social outlet that lifts the mood.

Be sure to inform class instructors of any arthritic modifications your doctor has recommended before beginning.

Balance Exercises

Some of the exercises already described in this book are wonderful for improving balance if you have arthritis. Balancing on one foot, walking heel-to-toe, leg raises, and hip exercises improve the strength and stability of the joints without causing unnecessary and painful impacts. Practicing these gentle balancing techniques will result in a growth of confidence and control. Be sure to use a chair, wall, or partner until you become more steady.

Walking

Walking is a perfect exercise for anyone to do with or without arthritis. It is low-impact, requires no training gym or equipment, and has a broad spectrum of benefits. Walking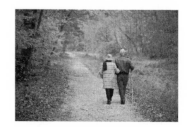

improves cardiovascular health, circulation of blood flow and oxygen to the muscles and joints, increases lung capacity, reduces instability, strengthens muscles, and releases endorphins for a wonderful lift in mood. Walking can also improve sleeping patterns and is very easy on the joints.

It's recommended to start slowly and walk with a partner. Having a partner to walk with is for safety measures, but it is also a great way to strengthen the bond of a relationship.

STRENGTH TRAINING

Strength training isn't only for the young and fit. It is an ideal way to build muscle mass which directly addresses the common condition of sarcopenia (or muscle loss) that happens when we age. The key is to start very slowly with small weights and work your way up as you get stronger. An eight-ounce or ten-ounce can of soup may be used before moving on to one pound weight if necessary. It is important to focus on the upper and lower body when strength training, and seek the assistance of a partner or friend when you begin. Muscle loss can result in frailness and osteoarthritis so building the muscles back up will counteract these effects.

Yoga

Yoga involves a gentle series of stretches and balance poses that increase circulation and flexibility. It delivers more oxygen to the joints and decreases swelling and pain, making it a stellar choice of exercise for someone with arthritis. It is best to perform this with an instructor and inform the instructor of the arthritic condition. Several modifications can be incorporated to improve the quality of benefits of exercising with yoga regularly.

Stretching

Dynamic stretching improves blood flow to the muscles, lubricates the joints, and warms the muscles for increased flexibility. It prepares the body for movement and decreases the chance of pulled muscles or falling. There are several stretches outlined in this book that can be done to ease joint pain if you have arthritis. Shoulder rolls, ankle and wrist rolls, arm swings, and stretching the calves and hamstrings can all contribute to reduced pain and increased stability.

* * *

SAMPLE ARTHRITIS-SAFE EXERCISE PLAN

Monday: Tai Chi, Balance Exercises

Tuesday: Pool Exercises, Walking

Wednesday: Strength Training, Walking

Thursday: Yoga, Balance Exercises

Friday: Stretching

Saturday: Tai Chi, Balance Exercises

Sunday: Stretching

EXERCISES SAFE FOR ARTHRITIS IN THE HANDS OR WRISTS

Fist-Close: Close the hand into a fist as best you can and hold for ten seconds. It's okay if the hand cannot completely close at first or it can only close for a few seconds. Practicing will increase the hand's flexibility and will help relieve tension. Repeat this exercise ten times a day.

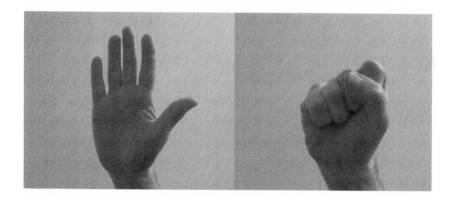

WRIST BENDS: WITH THE RIGHT ELBOW SUPPORTED ON A TABLE or pillow, take the left hand and slowly pull backward on the right hand to give the wrist a gentle stretch. Then, put the right hand down and push it down a bit more with the left hand. Hold for 30 seconds. Keep in mind that this stretch should not be done hard enough to cause pain, and it's okay if the hand doesn't bend very far at first. Switch hands and repeat the exercise. Repeat this exercise two times a day. Regular practice will lower stiffness and pain in the wrists.

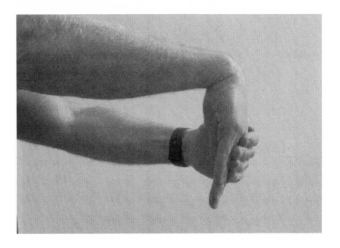

MAKE AN "O": ATTEMPT TO MAKE AN "O" WITH THE HAND BY touching the fingers around to the thumb. Hold for 30 seconds and repeat with the other hand. Perform this exercise five times a day. This might be very difficult in the beginning but should get easier with time and practice. It will help to loosen the hands by giving them a little stretch and delivering oxygen to the muscles and joints.

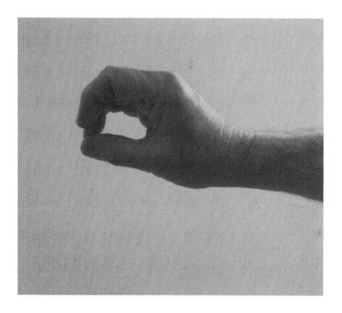

EXERCISES FOR ARTHRITIS IN THE HIPS OR KNEES

Sitting Stretch: Begin in the sitting position with the legs and feet supported and outstretched in front of you. The floor or a bed can be used for this exercise. Bend and stretch forward as though touching your toes. Be sure to move slowly and gently to receive the full benefits of the stretch in the hips and legs. Hold this pose for 30 seconds. With practice, the hips will become more flexible and stable.

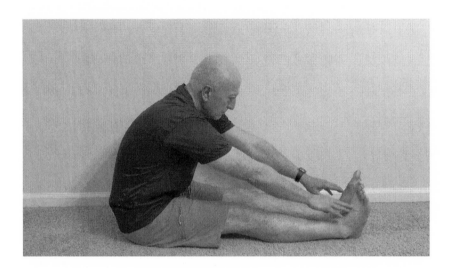

Step-Ups - Approach a set of stairs and hold on to the railing for support and balance. Step onto the first stair slowly and with control, then step back down. The gentle bend in the knee can help release tension and pain from arthritis. Repeat a few times a day alternating legs.

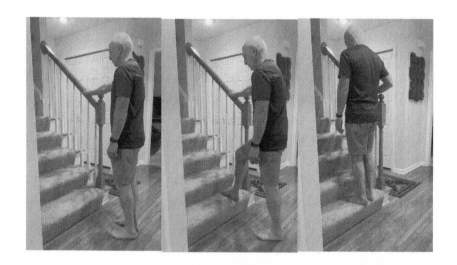

EXERCISES FOR ARTHRITIS IN THE ANKLES OR FEET

Ankle Circles: Utilize a chair or partner for support while lifting the foot and rotating it in a clockwise direction five times. Repeat five more circles but in the counterclockwise direction. Stretching the ankle relieves stress on the joints and lowers pain. Also, by reducing pain and stiffness, balance improves as well.

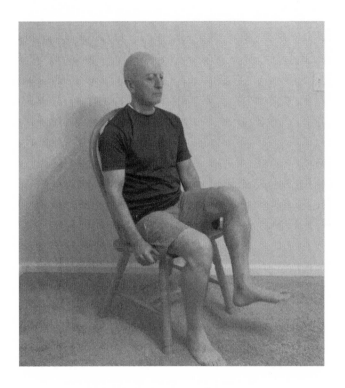

See videos of these exercises at www.betterbalanceforall.com

* * *

EXERCISES FOR ARTHRITIS IN MULTIPLE AREAS

Swimming: Swimming or joining a water aerobics class is ideal for people experiencing arthritis in multiple areas of the body. The water relieves physical and mental stress, increases endurance by working the heart and lungs, and improves mobility by strengthening the muscles. The gentleness fluidity of swimming exercises allows for considerably increased movements without exacerbating arthritic sensitivities.

Yoga or Tai Chi: Both yoga and tai chi focus on easy movements that provide gentle stretches and incorporate breathing techniques. Thoughtful control through the movements allows for improvement of flexibility and stability all while modifying for the comfort of the joints. Improving mobility in the joints using yoga and tai chi reduces pain and inflammation caused by arthritis.

EXERCISES FOR THOSE WITH LIMITED MOBILITY

Having limited mobility can reduce a person's confidence and discourage exercise. However, this doesn't have to be the case. Performing exercises that are designed to account for limited mobility can increase movement abilities and overall confidence. It is important to consider what types of exercise are best for someone with limited mobility and focus on those that will accommodate their physical needs. These exercises will increase energy levels, enhance mood, improve circulation, and maintain flexibility in the muscles and joints.

Cardiovascular Exercises: These exercises will give the heart a workout to improve the efficiency of each beat. Water aerobics is especially beneficial to those with limited mobility, because it reduces pain and stiffness in the joints as well. Dancing is another cardiovascular exercise that can be performed even if confined to a chair.

Strength Training Exercises: Lifting weights and building up muscle in the upper body is possible from a chair and provides an array of physical benefits. If the upper body has limited mobility then it is best to focus strength training on the legs and hips. Regardless, strengthening all muscles possible will result in a higher quality of life and better balance.

Flexibility Exercises: Stretching and performing other flexibility exercises are important especially if one is experiencing limited mobility. The exercises increase blood flow and keep the muscles from deteriorating further. They also relieve pain and increase joint mobility.

While thus far we've mostly discussed traditional exercise methods, the next chapter will delve into tai chi movements as an avenue for claiming back your vitality and balance. Explore the origins of tai chi, how to perform the movements, and why tai chi is especially beneficial to seniors. Making tai chi a regular practice will provide a plethora of positive physical results but it is also nurturing to our mind and mental state.

Continue to chapter eight to find out how tai chi can improve your overall quality of life, confidence, and stability.

8

PERFORMING TAI CHI MOVEMENTS

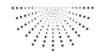

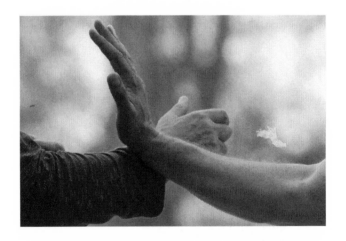

The ancient Chinese martial art, Tai Chi, helps seniors regain strength and improves their balance through a series of elegant movements. There are profound elements of stress relief and relaxation from each session. This chapter will explain all of the benefits of Tai Chi for seniors in detail as well as describe a few Tai Chi movements that are easy to follow.

TAI CHI FOR IMPROVED BALANCE

Tai Chi instructor, Stanwood Chang of the Benson-Henry Institute for Mind-Body Medicine, stated, "In just twelve weeks, I've seen people improve their balance and stability and walk faster and farther."

The fluid motions train the body how to breathe deeper and slower to reduce the anxiousness of the mind. One pose flows into the next in a graceful and controlled motion. While the weight and limbs change positions slowly, the muscles and joints compensate and engage accordingly. The result is what appears to be a graceful dance. Performing Tai Chi movements takes practice and dedicated effort. The outcome on the body from practicing Tai Chi is a stronger body, more flexible joints, controlled breathing, a calm mind, lower blood pressure, less cortisol (stress hormone) release, and an overall relaxation effect.

The balance improvements come from the particular movements that are done to stay upright during a session of Tai Chi. Transitioning from one pose to the next requires the muscles to elongate, engage, and compensate for the weight shift. There is a heightened awareness that is needed for staying balanced in the Tai Chi poses. Moving fluidly between them trains the mind to see obstacles, be conscientious of our surroundings, and know our body's capabilities. When we become more familiar with our bodies and how to move them to remain balanced, we can push ourselves to new levels of difficulty with a significantly lower risk of falling and a greater sense of confidence. Staying mindful of each motion in practice will train the mind to become more conscientious in everyday movements. Slow, confident, and purposeful motion is the key to balance improvement.

For seniors, Tai Chi is especially beneficial because it contributes to so much more than balance improvements. By having a heightened sense of awareness in the body, it is easier to predict what motions could inflame a joint or recover injury. If a movement becomes painful to do, it is detected sooner and can be modified to directly compensate for the troubled area of the body. Tai Chi also improves cognition which results in better memory recall.

Becoming stronger, more stable, increasing flexibility, and feeling in control are all effects of regular Tai Chi practice, and directly contribute to significantly reduced fear of falling. This martial art has the added benefit for seniors of easing arthritis pain. The slow and fluid motions help strengthen the joints and deliver more oxygen to the tissues. Tai Chi is a preferred exercise for people suffering from arthritis for all of these reasons, but in addition to the benefits listed, the gentleness of Tai Chi means that the exercises won't result in arthritic flare-ups.

It is recommended to speak with a doctor before starting a Tai Chi routine to be sure that any conditions are taken into consideration and proper modifications can be implemented. Also, if at any point one experiences dizziness or lightheadedness, stop and sit down immediately until symptoms subside.

As always, if you experience pain or dizzy episodes, consult your physician right away.

HOW TO DO TAI CHI

Warm-up

Leg Warm-Up: This warm-up can be performed using a chair for balance, with the hands resting on the hips, or arms comfortably down at your sides. Begin with a stance slightly wider than your shoulders and shift approximately 70% of your body weight to one leg while keeping both feet planted. Slowly shift weight onto the other leg and back again for at least three repetitions.

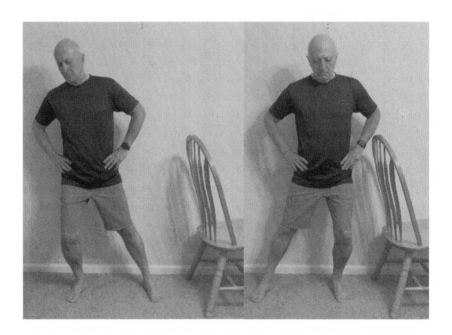

TORSO TWIST: AFTER THE LEG WARM-UP, PLACE YOUR HANDS on your waist and turn the upper body while keeping the hips square and stationary. Take a deep breath and lengthen the spine. Twist the torso just a bit further on the exhale focusing on the spine. Knees should be just slightly bent and knees should remain directly above the ankles. With the deeper twist, the hips may turn slightly but the twist should primarily remain in the spine. Keeping consciousness of where the twist is focused will naturally engage the core muscles and improve stability. Use slow and deep breaths to guide you in and out of the twist at least five times in each direction.

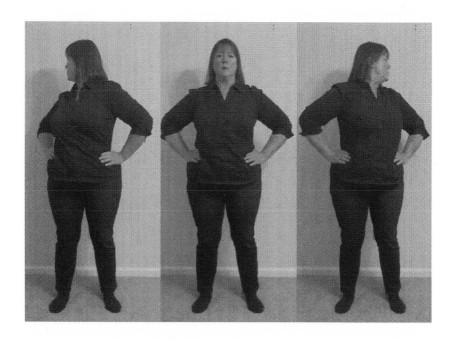

ENERGY TO THE SKY

This movement will originate from the core and back muscles while incorporating arm movements. Keeping focus and control while moving through the Energy to the Sky pose will contribute to digestion, breathing, and strengthening the engaged muscle groups.

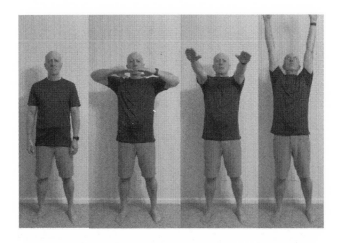

Begin the pose in the same neutral stance as those from the warm-up exercises, with the feet at a comfortable distance apart and the arms down at your sides. Raise your arms to shoulder height with the elbows bent and fingers facing in towards each other. Inhale deeply while straightening the elbows and extending the arms out with the palms facing downward. Pause and exhale while looking at your hands. Hold the gaze on the hands, and take another slow breath in while raising the arms straight above your head. Now exhale and bring your hands back down to your sides. Repeat the series of movements five times.

DRAWING THE BOW

Drawing the Bow engages muscles in the legs, shoulders, arms, and chest. Activating the chest with this series of motions will stimulate the heart and improve circulation throughout the body.

Starting with the right foot, step out just wider than the shoulders, and angle the head and torso to the right as well. The twist should mimic that of the torso twist in the warm-up. The hips should stay square to the feet while the spine twists. Close the hands into loose fists and reach them both out to the right. One arm will naturally reach further than the other in this twisted stance. Point the index finger and thumb of the right hand in an 'L' shape, keep your gaze just beyond your hands, and rotate the shoulders to point your imaginary arrow towards the sky. Simultaneously, draw the left elbow back and bend the knees into a squatting position upon exhaling. Then, take a slow breath in.

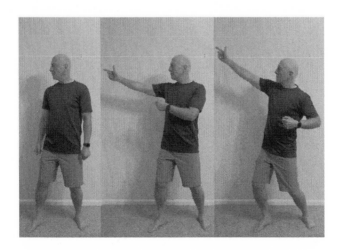

When you're ready to exhale again, use the breath to bring you back into a standing position with the torso facing forwards and your arms down comfortably at your sides. Drawing the Bow should be performed three times on each side.

Penetrating Heaven and Earth

The movements within Penetrating Heaven and Earth stretch the torso and stimulate circulation to the organs and joints. It provides a deep but gentle stretch to the shoulders as well.

Establish a sound base before starting these movements by placing the feet just wider than the width of your shoulders. The arms should be resting gently at the sides of the body. Start with the hands open and the palms facing inward. Draw the hands up with elbows bending out while inhaling deeply. The fingertips should meet at the chest and almost touch. Pause and exhale with the arms in this cradle-like position.

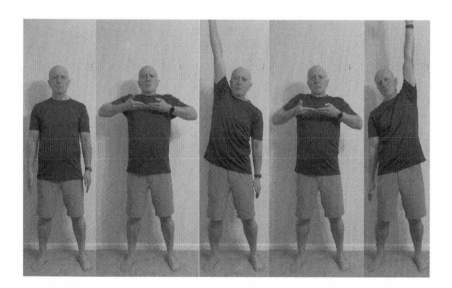

Then inhale again and send the right hand up with the palm pushing toward the sky. Simultaneously send the left hand down with the palm pushing toward the ground. Once fully extended, start the exhale while bringing both hands back to meet at the chest in the cradle-like position. Pause before inhaling and starting the arm extending motion again but with hands moving in opposite directions than before. Continue breathing slowly, move with control, and perform the motions eight times on each side. End the series of Penetrating Heaven and Earth by resting the hands and arms down comfortably at your sides again.

These are only a few of the many Tai Chi movement exercises. Tai Chi practitioners take years to master these movements. We recommend that for a more thorough understanding of Tai Chi exercises you register in a Tai Chi class, perhaps at your local Senior Citizens Center or local YMCA.

See videos of these exercises at www.betterbalanceforall.com

* * *

SAMPLE TAI CHI EXERCISE PLAN

Monday: Leg Warm-up, Torso Twist, Energy to the Sky, Drawing the Bow

Tuesday: Rest

Wednesday: Leg Warm-up, Torso Twist, Energy to the Sky, Penetrating Heaven and Earth

Thursday: Leg Warm-up, Torso Twist, Drawing the Bow, Penetrating Heaven and Earth

Friday: Rest

Saturday: Leg Warm-up, Torso Twist, Energy to the Sky, Drawing the Bow

Sunday: Rest

* * *

WHILE THIS SERIES OF TAI CHI EXERCISES OFFER A PLETHORA of benefits, starting a new exercise routine can produce some soreness and stiffness afterward. Experiencing the discomforts of muscle strengthening and stretching the joints can be discouraging, but it should not be debilitating.

If there is intolerable pain after an exercise, a physician should be consulted immediately. However, even with a tolerable amount of discomfort, it can be difficult to get excited about doing it all over again tomorrow. There may not be pain or discomfort immediately, but it can present itself after some time once the exercises are completed.

This is called *Delayed Onset Muscle Soreness (DOMS)*, and there are easy ways to remedy it that we'll outline in detail in the next chapter.

9

WHAT DOMS IS AND HOW TO DEAL WITH IT

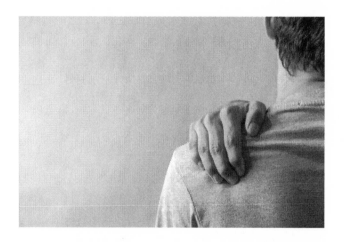

Experiencing pain up to a couple of days after exercising is not uncommon. It is referred to as Delayed Onset Muscle Soreness, or DOMS. Even though it can be expected that muscles will be a bit sore or stiff after a good workout, too much discomfort can discourage people from continuing a new exercise program. That is why we've put together some solutions to address DOMS. With the information and tools provided in this chapter, starting and maintaining a new exercise routine will be exciting and empowering.

It is simple to identify DOMS by the tell-tale symptoms.

The first sign that you're being affected by DOMS is that there is no pain during the workout and the soreness only presents itself a day or two later. The muscles will feel tired, weak, painful to touch, and sore when used. This happens when performing various high-intensity exercises but it is very typical after performing eccentric exercises.

An **eccentric exercise** requires the muscle to flex and lengthen at the same time. These types of exercises are found to cause micro-traumas to the muscle that are often only felt the next day. Believe it or not, there are benefits to experiencing the fallout from DOMS. The muscles repair the micro-traumas and recover with tissue that is better equipped to handle the stress of the exercise.

Anyone can experience DOMS, as it does not discriminate based on level of fitness. It can be the result of performing an exercise that the body isn't accustomed to or when the level of exercise is bumped up a notch. However, experiencing DOMS after an exercise routine is not an indicator that it was a 'good' workout. Beginning a new exercise routine is hard work and may result in muscle tenderness, but as the muscles get stronger, the soreness will not be as common after a workout. That does not mean that the body is getting less benefit from the exercises. It simply means that the muscles are getting stronger and adapting to the exertions.

HOW TO FIND RELIEF FROM DOMS

Several tools can be used to treat DOMS, but it is important to understand that they are not cures. The stiffness and soreness will take time to fully rectify. And, while waiting, these are the best treatments possible to ease the discomfort.

The symptoms of DOMS can tempt anyone to take on a couch-potato status until the pain is gone. But I assure you that taking that approach will only result in more pain and stiffness. It is best to keep moving so the muscles stay fluid. Several gentle movements will help keep the muscle warm and decrease the pain. Some exercises that have been covered in previous chapters are gentle enough to keep the muscles moving while recovering from DOMS such as yoga, tai chi, walking, and swimming. But we'll describe a selection of other treatment methods that can help ease the pain and stiffness considerably. Trying one or two methods and changing them up now and then will help you find what suits you best. We'll start with the massage.

Ten Minute Massage

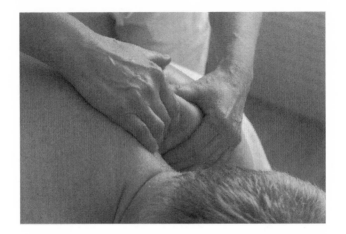

Massage is an effective treatment to reduce the pain and stiffness of DOMS, and can end up preventing it altogether. It is recommended that the most beneficial massage should be done 48 hours after a workout. This may not be possible or might be impractical if your exercise routine is four or five days a week. In that case, self-massage may be the best option.

Using an oil or lotion to work the muscles with your hands can have similar effects to professional massages. Spend ten minutes loosening the muscles by kneading and squeezing the muscles as well as giving them a gentle shake. Foam rollers can help to massage the muscles as well if there is a weakness or arthritic pain in the hands. Focus on the calves, glutes, thighs, arms, and shoulders. And by all means, schedule an appointment with a masseuse as often as you can. They have wonderful relaxing benefits, can help with sleep, and increase endorphin release in addition to treating DOMS.

Topical Analgesics

Topical analgesics are medicated balms that are absorbed into the skin for pain relief. Creams or gels with menthol in them will give the skin a warming or cooling sensation which distracts the brain from the pain. While this type of topical medication doesn't relieve the pain directly, some find it to be very effective at reducing the pain they are experiencing. Another type of topical agent that is often used for pain relief is those that contain capsaicin.

Capsaicin is the molecule that binds to the cells of our tongue from spicy peppers that creates the burning sensation. When it is applied to the skin over a sore muscle, the same type of effect happens. The skin and muscles feel warm and tingly. Another medication, *Arnica,* has anti-inflammatory properties, and when applied to the skin over a sore muscle, may provide some pain relief.

However, all of these medications can be dangerous if not used properly or if a person has an allergy or sensitivity to the ingredients. For that reason, be sure to consult your physician before using any topical medication, and wash your hands thoroughly after each application. Even with washed hands, avoid touching the eyes or any sensitive areas for several hours after applying the cream to a muscle. Though all topical creams mentioned have to be reapplied several times throughout a DOMS, they are still very helpful in giving some relief.

Cold Bath

Cold baths, commonly also known as ice baths, are used to treat muscle soreness by reducing the inflammation in the sore muscles. This happens through the constriction of the blood vessels which reduces the blood flow and swelling in a muscle. However, there are some important tips to keep in mind when using this form of pain relief.

If dipping into a cold water bath after vigorous exercise, the cold water will likely feel great and help with bringing the body's temperature down. Just be sure not to stay in the cold bath too long or the water will end up bringing your core temperature down too low, and that can be dangerous.

Ice baths are often used by athletes under the supervision of a physician, physical therapist, or coach. It isn't a bad idea to be sure that the same type of assistance is near when attempting a cold bath. It is recommended that when first starting this type of treatment, the **water shouldn't be any lower than 68-degrees Fahrenheit and not stay in the bath for longer than ten minutes**. The actual benefits of the cold bath wane after only two to three minutes so a shorter dip might be the best option. Be sure to consult a physician before attempting to use ice or cold baths as a treatment for muscle pain as they are dangerous for people with the following conditions: heart disease, high blood pressure, diabetes, peripheral neuropathy, poor circulation, venous stasis, or cold agglutinin disease. (Cleveland Clinic, 2022)

Warm Bath

For many people, a cold water bath does not sound very pleasant or appealing. In this case, a warm bathtub soak might be a better option for you. Keep in mind that there are appropriate times for taking a warm bath versus a cold bath with the biggest difference being that of their effects on blood flow.

While cold baths constrict the blood vessels, limiting blood flow, taking a warm bath opens them and has the opposite effect.

Taking a warm bath right after a new, or particularly intense, workout is beneficial in preventing and treating muscle soreness including that of DOMS.

However, the bath should be warm, rather than hot, so as not to burn the skin or shock the capillaries. When a warm bath is taken after a workout, it opens the blood vessels and allows for increased blood exchange in the muscle. More nutrients are delivered to the tissue and metabolic waste from the cells, such as lactic acid, is removed at a higher than normal rate. Improvements in muscle pain from DOMS of up to 47% when a warm bath is taken within 24 hours of exercising.

As always, consult an expert if you aren't sure whether a cold bath or a warm bath is more appropriate for your particular symptoms.

Warm baths do wonders for sore muscles, but they have the added benefit of being a source of stress relief as well. Several bath additives contribute to the relaxation effect of a warm bath such as essential oils, milk, oats, and fizzy bath bombs. If a warm bath isn't doable after exercise for you, try a warm wrap, heating blanket, or warm compress. These will all increase blood flow to the muscles as well. There are also several do-it-yourself tutorials online for how to make a microwavable heat pillow out of rice. This can be a great project to take on with a craft class or friend. They also make great gifts during the holidays.

Anti-Inflammatory Foods

While there isn't conclusive research just yet, there is supportive evidence of certain foods easing inflammation in the body which can in turn ease pain. Foods that are classified as an anti-inflammatory are outlined below.

Carbohydrates - Chia seed pudding, crackers, fruit, oatmeal, quinoa, rice cakes, sweet potatoes, whole grain bread, and whole grain cereal.

Protein - Chocolate milk, cottage cheese, eggs, Greek yogurt, turkey or chicken, salmon or tuna, peanut butter, protein shakes, and tofu scrambles.

Healthy fats - Avocado, coconut oil, flax seeds, nut butters, and nuts.

While this list of helpful treatment tips for improving DOMS symptoms is not all-inclusive, it is a great start for anyone seeking some relief. Try one treatment or any combination of them and we're sure you'll be feeling better in no time. However, there are a couple more notes to take on recovering from DOMS.

There is research that suggests anti-inflammatory medications don't provide much in terms of pain relief. So, no need to reach for Advil in the case of DOMS. Also, if you find that the soreness and stiffness are lasting longer than a week then it's time to consult a physician. Keep an eye out for any dark spots and swelling in the arms or legs. If any of these concerns are presenting themselves, seek medical treatment immediately.

Also talk to a doctor if you experience the muscle twitching or spasming, if the muscle becomes numb or starts to tingle, or if the pain goes from a dull ache to sudden sharp pain. And, of course, do not proceed with any exercise routine following any of these mentioned symptoms without getting clearance to do so from your physician.

There are a few ways that may assist with avoiding DOMS entirely. They are not fool-proof but they can help and are considered best-practice to avoid injury. Firstly, drink plenty of water. Warm-up before exercising using the dynamic exercises provided in this book. Cool down for about 20 minutes after an exercise with static exercises, some easy cycling, or low-intensity strength training. And lastly, exercise at a comfortable level of difficulty for you. Don't amp up the intensity of a workout until you're ready. Allow the muscles to adjust to new exercises before taking them to the next level.

Everyone will have a slightly different pace that their body is happy with. It is important to listen to what the body is telling us and adjust accordingly.

CONCLUSIONS

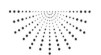

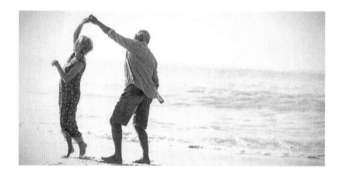

There are so many memories to be made and experiences to be had in the senior years. No need to miss out on fun with the grandkids building a garden, taking long walks, going on vacations, or attending school functions.

Without fear of falling, true happiness awaits you and those you love. Building up a stronger and more capable body means regaining a level of independence and a sense of accomplishment. Your peers, family members, and community will benefit from the beautiful source of confidence you provide after completing a new exercise program and maintaining the new you. Getting through daily tasks without muscle weakness, instability, or fear is a direct result of hard work and dedication. The exercises provided in this book are only one part of the solution for fearlessness. The other requirement to achieving greater balance in 28 days is the sheer willpower to do the work.

The various exercises and stretches provided in this book were specifically chosen for their contributions to the approach known as **SMM, or stretching, mobility training,** and **strength training**. This approach addresses the many factors that contribute to the fear of falling including muscle weakness, loss of bone density, muscle stiffness, inner ear issues, and more. The goal is to identify what potential problems someone could be facing when it comes to a reluctance of physical activity, and offer tools to break down the physical and mental obstacles standing in the way. Achieving a new state of confidence and stability is possible for anyone.

This book is intended for senior citizens living all sorts of lifestyles. It gives options to customize a 28-day plan that will work best with those different lifestyles in mind. If mobility is limited, and living arrangements include an assisted living facility, then exercises can be modified to accommodate. An individual's abilities and the tools a facility has to offer should be taken into consideration and adjusted accordingly. If an individual lives at home alone, or with a spouse, suggestions for using what is available at home are included in this book as well. Regardless of circumstance, there are options that anyone can benefit from.

While *Never Fear Falling Again* is designed to give you options of what might work best for you initially, it can also be used to maintain your newfound stability and strengthen your body even further. For example, if you are struggling with vertigo and muscle weakness as your main contributor to a loss of balance, then you can work through this book in stages. The initial 28 days might consist of vertigo exercises and chair exercises. Using the weekly exercise plans suggested in chapters two and six will help get you strong enough to move on to standing exercises and Tai Chi practice. Whatever level you may be starting at, there is an appropriate approach to addressing the main culprits of your instability and fears.

It is important to remember to stay as consistent as possible with the workout plans and do not give up. Occasionally, setbacks happen. That's okay! We all have them at times. However, coming back to a regular exercise routine is the best thing you can do to regain a sense of confidence and normality. If the routine needs to change a bit to accommodate new physical circumstances, that's okay too. Remember that every exercise completed will only make you stronger.

If you find that life is busy and your social calendar is getting in the way of your workout plan then it may be time to consider merging the two. Ask a friend or family member to share a walk or new yoga class with you. Exercising can be a wonderful bonding opportunity for loved ones to enjoy together. Even just a quick grapevine in the kitchen to your favorite song will get the grandkids moving along with you. Also, if exercising is made a priority in your life then you can count on being more physically able to join in on social events for years to come.

Use *Never Fear Falling Again* as a menu of exercise options that will start as a 28-day program, but give you lifelong options to maintain the balance and confidence that is built. Each person will have slightly different needs, so listen to your body and choose a plan that is achievable but challenges you to improve your quality of life.

Day after day, you will wake up feeling a bit stronger and a bit more capable than you were the day before. Progress will be gradual so taking notes as you go along might be helpful to see how far you've come. However, there will inevitably come the day when you realize you'd never have had the confidence to do *that* 28 days ago.

So, take the step, do the stretch, complete the set, and get on your way to the sense of balance and confidence that waits.

Wake up excited for the day again. Say "yes" to the seniors' social gathering; go on the next family vacation!

A whole new perspective on life awaits you.

REFERENCES

Authors, E. (2019, October 9). *Core exercises for seniors to strengthen muscles and prevent falls.* Elizz. https://elizz.-com/wellness/core-exercises-for-seniors/

Barlas, P., Craig, J. A., Robinson, J., Walsh, D. M., Baxter, G. D., & Allen, J. M. (2000). Managing delayed-onset muscle soreness: Lack of effect of selected oral systemic analgesics. *Archives of Physical Medicine and Rehabilitation,* 81(7), 966–972. https://doi.org/10.1053/apmr.2000.6277

Best exercise for balance: Tai chi. (2014, December 6). Harvard Health. https://www.health.harvard.edu/staying-healthy/best-exercise-for-balance-tai-chi#:~:text=Tai%20chi%20is%20an%20ancient

Bubnis, D. (2019, June 3). *Tai chi moves: How to get started, benefits, seniors, and more.* Healthline. https://www.health-line.com/health/exercise-fitness/tai-chi-moves#benefits

Capritto, A. (2019, September 1). *Should you use heat or ice for sore muscles?* CNET. https://www.cnet.com/health/fit-ness/is-hot-or-cold-better-for-sore-muscles/

Coe, C. (2020, August 5). 7 *Causes of balance issues in the golden years.* Home Care Assistance of Jefferson County. https://www.homecareassistancejeffersonco.com/what-can-be-causing-my-elderly-parents-balance-difficulties/

Contributors, W. E. (2021, March 18). *What causes balance issues in older adults.* WebMD. https://www.webmd.com/healthy-aging/what-causes-balance-issues-in-older-adults

Davidson, K. (2020, July 20). *Arnica homeopathic medicine: overview, uses, and benefits.* Healthline. https://www.healthline.com/nutrition/arnica-homeopathic

Fraticelli, T. (2019, May 19). 12 *Balance exercises for seniors | with printable pictures and PDF.* PTProgress | Career Development, Education, Health. https://www.ptprogress.com/balance-exercises-for-seniors/

Healthwise, S. (2020, December 2). *Vertigo: balance exercises |* Michigan Medicine. Www.uofmhealth.org. https://www.uofmhealth.org/health-library/ug1239

Home, K. at. (2016, December 7). *Balance disorders in older adults: 3 important things to know.* Www.kendalathome.org. https://www.kendalathome.org/blog/balance-disorders-in-older-adults

Khanna, T. (2020, November 12). *How seniors can maintain flexibility through stretching.* The Physio Co. https://www.thephysioco.com.au/the-benefits-of-stretching-for-seniors/

Kilroy, D. (2014, September 8). *Exercise plan for seniors: strength, stretching, and balance.* Healthline. https://www.healthline.com/health/everyday-fitness/senior-workouts#Exercise-plan-for-seniors

Kimbrell, J. (2022, February 28). *7 Gentle exercises for seniors with arthritis*. A Place for Mom. https://www.aplaceformom.-com/caregiver-resources/articles/gentle-exercises-for-seniors-with-arthritis

Kutcher, M. (2019, July 19). *Soreness after exercise or physical activity* | More Life Health. More Life Health - Seniors Health & Fitness. https://morelifehealth.com/articles/doms#:~:text=If%20you%20have%20found%20yourself

Lambden, D. (2017, November 6). *Inner ear balance exercises*. Clear Living. https://www.clearliving.com/hearing/hearing-loss/inner-ear-balance-exercises/

McIntyre, K. (2022, January 7). *5 Balance exercises that can help prevent falls*. Lifemark. https://www.lifemark.ca/blog-post/5-balance-exercises-can-help-prevent-falls

Mills, M. (2020, January 28). *18 Chair exercises for seniors & how to get started*. Vive Health. https://www.vivehealth.-com/blogs/resources/chair-exercises-for-seniors

Olson, G. (2019, June 25). *What is delayed onset muscle soreness (DOMS) and what can you do about it?* Healthline; Healthline Media. https://www.healthline.com/health/doms

Orenstein, B. (2020, March 26). *7 Fall prevention exercises for people with arthritis*. EverydayHealth.com. https://www.everydayhealth.com/arthritis-pictures/fall-prevention-exercises-for-people-with-arthritis.aspx

Orthopaedics. (2022, March 21). *Brrr! What ice baths can do for sore muscles.* Cleveland Clinic. https://health.cleveland-clinic.org/can-ice-baths-ease-my-sore-muscles/

Pathak, N. (2021, August 30). *Topical pain relief: creams, gels, and rubs.* WebMD. https://www.webmd.com/pain-management/topical-pain-relievers

Poor circulation treatment & causes | Center for Vascular Medicine. (n.d.). Www.cvmus.com. https://www.cvmus.com/vascular-treatment/poor-circulation-treatment-and-causes

Radcliffe, S. (2019, January 3). *Exercise and best foods to aat afterward.* Healthline. https://www.healthline.com/health-news/what-are-the-best-foods-to-eat-after-an-intense-workout

Robinson, L. (2019). HelpGuide.org. HelpGuide.org. https://www.helpguide.org/articles/healthy-living/exercise-and-fitness-as-you-age.htm

The 10-minute stretching routine seniors should do daily. (2020, August 28). Careasone Blog. https://careasone.-com/blog/the-10-minute-stretching-routine-seniors-should-do-daily/

10 balance exercises for seniors that you can do at home. Balance Exercises for Seniors That You Can Do at Home. (2020, July 17). Snug Safety. https://www.snugsafe.com/all-posts/balance-exercises-for-seniors

21 Chair exercises for seniors: complete visual guide - California mobility. (2018, December 14). California Mobility. https://californiamobility.com/21-chair-exercises-for-seniors-visual-guide/

Vestibular_exercises. (n.d.). University of Mississippi Medical Center. https://www.umc.edu/Healthcare/ENT/Patient-Handouts/Adult/Otology/Vestibular_Exercises.html

Walker, O. (2019, April 3). *Post-exercise stretching | science for sport.* Science for Sport. https://www.scienceforsport.com/post-exercise-stretching/

Why Senior Citizens Should Perform Balance Exercises. (2020, June 24). Www.freedomcareny.com. https://www.freedomcareny.com/posts/why-should-senior-citizens-perform-balance-exercises

Williams, L. (2020, March 25). 11 Accessible Chair Exercises for Older Adults. Verywell Fit. https://www.verywellfit.com/chair-exercises-for-seniors-4161267

IMAGE REFERENCES

No-longer-here. (Nov. 1, 2017). *Zen stones pile.* [2907290] Pixabay. https://pixabay.com/photos/zen-stones-pile-stack-meditation-2907290/

HeikeFrohnhoff. (July 11, 2014). *Massage shoulder relaxing massage.* [389716] Pixabay. https://pixabay.com/photos/massage-shoulder-relaxing-massage-389716/

Kampfkunstbewegung. (Oct. 14, 2021). *Hands martial arts qi gong taiji.* [6706782] Pixabay. https://pixabay.com/photos/hands-martial-arts-qi-gong-taiji-6706782/

Psychonsultants. (June 2, 2021) *Woman adult yoga zen meditate.* [6304184] Pixabay. https://pixabay.com/photos/woman-adult-yoga-zen-meditate-6304184/

3534679. (Aug. 20, 2017) *Yoga calm release stretching.* [2662234] Pixabay. https://pixabay.com/photos/yoga-calm-release-stretching-2662234/

Sabinevanerp. (Sept. 11, 2018) *Hand woman grown up hands elderly.* [3667030] Pixabay. https://pixabay.com/photos/hand-woman-grown-up-hands-elderly-3667030/

Sabinevanerp. (Nov. 1, 2017) *Hand hands old old age ipad.* [2906425] Pixabay. https://pixabay.com/photos/hand-hands-old-old-age-ipad-2906425/

Pexels. (Nov. 23, 2016) *Feet legs swimming pool submerged.* [1853291] Pixabay. https://pixabay.com/photos/feet-legs-swimming-pool-submerged-1853291/

EddieKphoto. (Sept. 26, 2021) *Couple elderly walking fall trail.* [6653517] Pixabay. https://pixabay.com/photos/couple-elderly-walking-fall-trail-6653517/